GUIDE TO THE
LITERATURE FOR THE
INDUSTRIAL MICROBIOLOGIST

GUIDE TO THE
LITERATURE FOR THE
INDUSTRIAL MICROBIOLOGIST

Compiled by

Peter A. Hahn

IFI/PLENUM • NEW YORK-WASHINGTON-LONDON

Library of Congress Cataloging in Publication Data

Hahn, Peter A
  Guide to the literature for the industrial microbiologist.

  1. Industrial microbiology—Bibliography. I. Title. [DNLM: 1. Microbiology—
Bibliography. ZQW75 H148g 1960-73]
Z5180.H34   660'.62   73-19782
ISBN 0-306-68431-4

© 1973 IFI/Plenum Data Corporation
A Subsidiary of Plenum Publishing Corporation
227 West 17th Street, New York, N.Y. 10011

United Kingdom edition published by Plenum Press, London
A Division of Plenum Publishing Company, Ltd.
Davis House (4th Floor), 8 Scrubs Lane, Harlesden, London, NW10 6SE, England

Printed in the United States of America

FOREWORD

By 1960 the scientific community began observing
an ever increasing explosion in the literature embrac-
ing the many facets of industrial microbiology. Many
of the so-called traditional areas were being replaced
by more modern provocative channels of endeavor. It
was about this time that excellent review-type annual
publications, such as Advances in Applied Microbiology,
Progress in Industrial Microbiology and Developments
in Industrial Microbiology emerged reporting the ex-
citing new work. It was soon, thereafter, that the
Division of Microbial Chemistry shed its probationary
status to become a bona fide unit of the American Chemical Society. A rash of new applied microbiological

textbooks arrived on the scene. The number of journals
reporting the day-to-day scientific achievements also
burgeoned.

Early in my industrial career, I found it imperative to devise a "workable" key to the ever increasing
volume of literature that was emerging. This I compiled over the years on voluminous stacks of file cards
which have in essence been reprinted here as "my"
Guide to the Literature for the Industrial Microbiologist.
The Guide has, indeed, served me well and through it,
one can readily ascertain the state of the art of any
of the many specialized subjects of industrial microbiology.

Logically, one would first consult recent textbooks
to obtain an overview of the subject being searched.
In Section I, I have included the title and contents of
98 of the more relevant textbooks published in the area
of industrial microbiology -- many of which I have per-
sonally used and found to be most helpful.

Without a doubt, the most useful section of the
book is Section II - a guide to the review literature in
industrial microbiology with its some 1697 entries.
The review type articles included in the guide are ar-

ranged chronologically under fifty-seven broad subject headings. Not only does each review article give one a historical development of the subject being searched, but is followed by an exhaustive bibliography of the papers and patents cited from whence one might "dig deeper."

In order to keep abreast of the research being reported on in one's area of speciality it is, of course, imperative that one acquaint himself with specific papers as they appear in the current literature. Section III contains a listing of 30 of the more prominant journals and abstracting services available to the industrial microbiologist.

Attending annual meetings and refresher courses, too, help keep one's finger on the state of the art. The more important ones are given in Section IV.

The Guide essentially includes that literature generated between 1960 and mid 1973. My file cards, however, will continue to log in new entries with time which will, hopefully, find themselves some day in a new expanded and updated Guide to the Literature for the Industrial Microbiologist.

CONTENTS

SECTION I - INDUSTRIAL MICROBIOLOGICAL TEXTBOOKS

This section contains the title and contents of 98 of the more relevant textbooks published in the field of industrial microbiology. All but 12 of the books have been published since 1960.

ACTINOMYCETALES: CHARACTERISTICS AND PRACTICAL IMPORTANCE
Society for Applied Bacteriology Symposium Series #2
1973. Academic Press, N. Y. (356 pp.)

General Consideration and Implications of the Actinomycetales
Taxonomy and Classification of the Actinomycetes
The Fine Structure of the Actinomycetales
Genetics of the Actinomycetales
The Streptomyces Spore: Its Distinct Features and Germinal Behavior
Endospores of Actinomycetes: Dormancy and Germination
Secondary Metabolism with Special Reference to Actinomycetales
The Occurrence and Significance of Actinomycetes
Actinomycetes in Soils, Composts and Fodders
Streptomyces Scabies and Potato Scab Disease
Farmers' Lung Disease
Commensal and Pathogenic Actinomycetes in Man
The Significance of Bifidobacteria in the Intestinal Tract of Infants
A Rapid Method for the Identification of Bifidobacterium Species using 50 Characters

ACTINOMYCETES, THE - VOL. 1 (NATURE, OCCURRENCE, AND ACTIVI-
TIES) - S. A. Waksman. 1959. Williams and Wilkins Co., Baltimore (327 pp.)

Chapter	Contents	Page
1	Historical Background	1
2	Isolation, Identification, Cultivation and Preservation	17

Chapter	Contents	Page

ACTINOMYCETES, THE - VOL. 2 (CLASSIFICATION, IDENTIFICATION AND DESCRIPTIONS OF GENERA AND SPECIES) - S. A. Waksman. 1961. Williams and Wilkins Co., Baltimore (363 pp.)

Chapter	Contents	Page

ACTINOMYCETES, THE - VOL. 3 (ANTIBIOTICS OF ACTINOMYCETES) -
S. A. Waksman and H. A. Lechevalier. 1962. Williams and
Wilkins Co., Baltimore (430 pp.)

ACTINOMYCETES, THE - A SUMMARY OF CURRENT KNOWLEDGE - S. A.
Waksman. 1967. Ronald Press, N. Y. (280 pp.)

ANAEROBE LABORATORY MANUAL - L. V. Holdeman and W. E. C.
  Moore.   1972.   V. P. I. Anaerobe Lab., Blacksburg, Va.
  (130 pp.)

Contents   Page

AUTOMATION MECHANISM AND DATA HANDLING IN MICROBIOLOGY -
  A. Baillie, Editor, and R. J. Gilbert. 1970. Society
  for Applied Bacteriology Technical Series #4. Academic
  Press, N. Y. (248 pp.)

BACTERIA, THE - VOL. 1 (STRUCTURE) - Edited by I. C.
  Gunsalus and R. Y. Stanier. 1960. Academic Press, N. Y.
  (513 pp.)

Chapter   Contents   Page

BACTERIA, THE - VOL. 2 (METABOLISM) - Edited by I. C.
  Gunsalus and R. Y. Stanier. 1961. Academic Press, N. Y.
  (572 pp.)

Chapter   Contents   Page

Chapter	Contents	Page

BACTERIA, THE - VOL. 3 (BIOSYNTHESIS) - Edited by I. C. Gunsalus & R. Y. Stanier. 1962. Academic Press, N. Y. (718 pp.)

Chapter	Contents	Page

BACTERIA, THE - VOL. 4 (PHYSIOLOGY OF GROWTH) - Edited by
I. C. Gunsalus & R. Y. Stanier. 1962. Academic Press,
N. Y. (459 pp.)

BACTERIA, THE - VOL. 5 (HEREDITY) - Edited by I. C. Gunsalus
& R. Y. Stanier. 1964. Academic Press, N. Y.

BACTERIAL PHYSIOLOGY AND METABOLISM - J. R. Sokatch. 1969
Academic Press, N. Y.

Chapter	Contents	Page

BACTERIOLOGICAL ANALYTICAL MANUAL - U. S. Department of Health, Education and Welfare. Jan. 1969. Public Health Service, Food & Drug Administration, Field Scientific Coordination Staff, Washington, D. C. 2nd Edition.

Chapter	Contents

BERGEY'S MANUAL OF DETERMINATIVE BACTERIOLOGY - 7th Edition,
  1957. Williams and Wilkins Co., Baltimore, Md.

"An Elaborate System of Classification of Bacteria into
  Families, Tribes and Genera."

BIOCHEMICAL & BIOLOGICAL ENGINEERING SCIENCE - VOL. 1
  Edited by N. Blakebrough. 1967. Academic Press, N. Y.

Chapter   Contents

BIOCHEMICAL ENGINEERING - S. Aiba, A. E. Humphrey, N. F.
  Millis. 1965. Academic Press, N. Y. (333 pp.)

                         Contents   Page

BIOCHEMICAL ENGINEERING - R. Steel. 1958. The Macmillan
   Company, N. Y. (328 pp.)

Contents   Page

BIOCHEMICAL ENGINEERING - F. C. Webb. 1964. D. Van
   Nostrand Company, Great Britain (743 pp.)

Contents   Page

Contents   Page

BIOCHEMISTRY OF INDUSTRIAL MICRO-ORGANISMS - Edited by
   C. Rainbow and A. H. Rose.   1963.   Academic Press, N. Y.
   (708 pp.)

Chapter	Contents	Page

BIOSYNTHESIS OF ANTIBIOTICS - VOL. 1 - Edited by J. F. Snell.
   1966.   Academic Press, N. Y.

Chapter	Contents	Page

CHEMICALS FROM FERMENTATION - P. A. Hahn. 1968. Doubleday
    & Co., Garden City, N. Y. (112 pp.)

CONTINUOUS CULTIVATION OF MICROORGANISMS - Edited by I.
    Malek, K. Beran and J. Hospodka. 1964. Proceedings of
    the 2nd Symposium held in Prague, 1962. Academic Press,
    N. Y. (391 pp.)

41 papers on various aspects.

DIFCO MANUAL OF DEHYDRATED CULTURE MEDIA AND REAGENTS FOR
    MICROBIOLOGICAL AND CLINICAL LABORATORY PROCEDURES -
    9th Edition. 1953. Difco Laboratories, Detroit, Mich.
    (350 pp.)

ENZYME ENGINEERING - L. B. Wingard, Editor. 1972. Inter-
    science Publishers (Division of John Wiley and Sons, N. Y.)
    (415 pp.)

FERMENTATION ADVANCES - Edited by D. Perlman. 1969. (Proceedings of the III International Fermentation Symposium) Academic Press, N. Y. (909 pp.)

FERMENTATION TECHNOLOGY TODAY - Edited by Dr. Gyozo Terui. 1973. (Proceedings of the IVth International Fermentation Symposium) Society of Fermentation Technology, Japan (900 pp.)

<table>

Contents	Page

FUNGAL METABOLITES - W. B. Turner. 1971. Academic Press, N. Y. (446 pp.)

FUNGI, THE - VOL. 1 (THE FUNGAL CELL) - Edited by G. C.
  Aimsworth and Alfred S. Sussman. 1965. Academic Press,
  N. Y.

FUNGI, THE - VOL. 2 (THE FUNGAL ORGANISM) - Edited by G. C.
  Aimsworth and Alfred S. Sussman. 1966. Academic Press,
  N. Y.

FUNGI, THE - VOL. 3 (THE FUNGAL POPULATION) - Edited by
  G. C. Aimsworth and Alfred S. Sussman. 1968. Academic
  Press, N. Y.

GENETICS OF BACTERIA AND THEIR VIRUSES, THE - W. Hayes.
  1964. John Wiley and Sons, N. Y. (740 pp.)

GENUS ASPERGILLUS, THE - K. B. Raper and D. I. Fennell.
1965. Williams and Wilkins Co., Baltimore (686 pp.)

PART I - General Discussion

GLOBAL IMPACTS OF APPLIED MICROBIOLOGY - Editor M. P. Starr.
1964. Conference held in Stockholm, 1963. John Wiley &
Sons, N. Y. (572 pp.)

GUIDE TO THE CLASSIFICATION AND IDENTIFICATION OF THE AC-
TINOMYCETES AND THEIR ANTIBIOTICS - S. A. Waksman and
H. A. Lechevalier. 1953. Williams and Wilkins Co.,
Baltimore (246 pp.)

GUIDE TO THE IDENTIFICATION OF THE GENERA OF BACTERIA -
V. B. D. Skerman. 1967. 2nd Edition. Williams and
Wilkins Co., Baltimore.

HANDBOOK OF MICROBIOLOGY - VOL. 1 (ORGANISMIC MICROBIOLOGY) -
1973. Chemical Rubber Co., Cleveland, Ohio.

HANDBOOK OF MICROBIOLOGY - VOL. 2 (MICROBIAL COMPOSITION) -
Publication Due 1973. Chemical Rubber Co., Cleveland,
Ohio.

HANDBOOK OF MICROBIOLOGY - VOL. 3 (MICROBIAL PRODUCTS) -
Publication Due 1973. Chemical Rubber Co., Cleveland,
Ohio.

HANDBOOK OF MICROBIOLOGY - VOL. 4 (MICROBIAL METABOLISM,
GENETICS AND IMMUNOLOGY) - Publication Due 1973. Chemical
Rubber Co., Cleveland, Ohio.

IDENTIFICATION METHODS FOR MICROBIOLOGISTS (PART A) - Edited
by B. M. Gibbs and F. A. Skinner. 1966. Society for
Applied Bacteriology Technical Series #1. Academic Press,
N. Y.

Contents

IDENTIFICATION METHODS FOR MICROBIOLOGISTS (PART B) - Edited
by B. M. Gibbs and D. A. Shapton. 1968. Society for
Applied Bacteriology Technical Series #2. Academic Press,
N. Y.

Contents

Contents   Page

INDUSTRIAL FERMENTATIONS - VOL. 1 - L. A. Underkofler and
R. J. Hickey. 1954. Chemical Publishing Co., N. Y. (565
pp.)
Chapter   Contents   Page

INDUSTRIAL FERMENTATIONS - VOL. 2 - L. A. Underkofler and
R. J. Hickey. 1954. Chemical Publishing Co., N. Y. (578
pp.)
Chapter   Contents   Page

INDUSTRIAL MICROBIOLOGY - L. E. Casida, Jr. 1968. John Wiley and Sons, N. Y. (460 pp.)

PART I - Introduction

PART II - Basis & Development of Industrial Fermentation Processes

INDUSTRIAL MICROBIOLOGY - S. C. Prescott, C. G. Dunn. 1959. Third Edition, McGraw-Hill Book Company, N. Y. (945 pp.)

Contents

INTRODUCTION TO BACTERIAL PHYSIOLOGY, AN - E. Oginsky and
W. Umbreit. 1959. 2nd Edition. W. H. Freeman & Co.,
San Francisco (443 pp.)

SECTION ONE: The Nature of Bacterial Physiology

SECTION TWO: Bacterial Anatomy

INTRODUCTION TO INDUSTRIAL STERILIZATION - J. W. Richards.
  1968. Academic Press, N. Y. (183 pp.)

ISOLATION OF ANAEROBES - Editor D. A. Shapton and R. G. Board. 1971. Society for Applied Bacteriology Technical Series #5. Academic Press, N. Y. (284 pp.)

ISOLATION METHODS FOR MICROBIOLOGY - Editor D. A. Shapton and G. W. Gould. 1969. Society for Applied Bacteriology Technical Series #3. Academic Press, N. Y. (190 pp.)

LABORATORY METHODS IN MICROBIOLOGY - W. F. Harrigan and Margaret E. McCance. 1966. Academic Press, N. Y.

LIST OF FUNGAL PRODUCTS - S. Shibata, S. Natori and S. Udagawa. 1964. University of Tokyo Press, Tokyo. (170 pp.)

MANUAL OF CLINICAL MICROBIOLOGY - John E. Blair, Edwin
H. L. Lennette, and Joseph P. Truant. 1970. American
Society for Microbiology, Bethesda, Md.

MANUAL OF MICROBIOLOGICAL METHODS (SAM) - 1957. McGraw
Hill Book Company, N. Y. (315 pp.)

MANUAL OF THE PENICILLIA, A - K. B. Raper and C. Thom.
1949. Williams and Wilkins Company, Baltimore, Md. (875
pp.)

PART I - General Discussion

MATERIALS AND METHODS IN FERMENTATION - G. L. Solomons.
1969. Academic Press, N. Y. (331 pp.)

METHODS IN IMMUNOLOGY AND IMMUNOCHEMISTRY - VOL. 1 (PREPARA-
TION OF ANTIGENS AND ANTIBODIES) - Edited by Curtis A.
Williams and Merrill W. Chase. 1967. Academic Press,
N. Y. (479 pp.)

METHODS IN IMMUNOLOGY AND IMMUNOCHEMISTRY - VOL. 2 (PHYSICAL
AND CHEMICAL METHODS) - Edited by Curtis A. Williams and
Merrill W. Chase. 1968. Academic Press, N. Y.

METHODS IN IMMUNOLOGY AND IMMUNOCHEMISTRY - VOL. 3 - Edited
by Curtis A. Williams and Merrill W. Chase. 1970.
Academic Press, N. Y.

METHODS IN IMMUNOLOGY AND IMMUNOCHEMISTRY - VOL. 4 - Edited
by Curtis A. Williams and Merrill W. Chase. Academic
Press, N. Y.

METHODS IN MICROBIOLOGY - VOL. 1 - Edited by J. R. Norris
and D. W. Ribbons. 1969. Academic Press, N. Y.

METHODS IN MICROBIOLOGY - VOL. 2 - Edited by J. R. Norris
and D. W. Ribbons. 1970. Academic Press, N. Y.

METHODS IN MICROBIOLOGY - VOL. 3A - Edited by J. R. Norris
and D. W. Ribbons. 1970. Academic Press, N. Y.

METHODS IN MICROBIOLOGY - VOL. 3B - Edited by J. R. Norris and D. W. Ribbons. 1970. Academic Press, N. Y.

METHODS IN MICROBIOLOGY - VOL. 4 - Edited by J. R. Norris and D. W. Ribbons. 1971. Academic Press, N. Y.

METHODS IN MICROBIOLOGY - VOL. 5A - Edited by J. R. Norris
and D. W. Ribbons.   1971.   Academic Press, N. Y.

METHODS IN MICROBIOLOGY - VOL. 5B - Edited by J. R. Norris
and D. W. Ribbons. 1971. Academic Press, N. Y.

METHODS IN MICROBIOLOGY - VOL. 6A - Edited by J. R. Norris
and D. W. Ribbons. 1971. Academic Press, N. Y.

METHODS IN MICROBIOLOGY - VOL. 6B - Edited by J. R. Norris and D. W. Ribbons. 1972. Academic Press, N. Y.

METHODS IN MICROBIOLOGY - VOL. 7A - Edited by J. R. Norris and D. W. Ribbons. 1972. Academic Press, N. Y.

METHODS IN MICROBIOLOGY - VOL. 7B - Edited by J. R. Norris and D. W. Ribbons. 1972. Academic Press, N. Y.

MICROBIAL ASPECTS OF POLLUTION - Edited by G. Sykes and F. A. Skinner. 1971. Society for Applied Bacteriology Symposium Series #1. Academic Press, N. Y. (304 pp.)

Contents

Contents

Nitrogen Removal from Waste Waters by Biological Nitrifi-
cation and Denitrification
Degradation of Herbicides by Soil Microorganisms
The Microbial Breakdown of Pesticides
Biodeterioration and Biodegradation of Synthetic Polymes
Disposal of Infective Laboratory Materials

MICROBIAL TECHNOLOGY - Edited by H. J. Peppler. 1967.
   Reinhold Publishing Company, N. Y. (454 pp.)

MICROBIAL TOXINS - VOL. I (BACTERIAL PROTEIN TOXINS) -
   Edited by S. J. Ajl, S. Kadis and T. C. Montie.
   Academic Press, N. Y.

Chapter	Contents
6	Relationship of Lysogeny to Bacterial Toxin Production
7	Role of Toxins in Host-Parasite Relationships
8	Tissue Culture and Bacterial Protein Toxins
9	Pharmacology of Bacterial Protein Toxins
10	Relative Toxicities and Assay Systems
11	Immunology of Bacterial Protein Toxins
12	Relationship of Bacterial Structure and Metabolism to Toxin Production
13	Uptake of Bacterial Protein Toxins by Cells

MICROBIAL TOXINS - VOL. IIA (BACTERIAL PROTEIN TOXINS) -
Edited by S. Kadis, T. C. Montie and S. J. Ajl.
Academic Press, N. Y.

Chapter	Contents
1	Botulinum Toxin
2	Tetanus Toxin
3	Type A Clostridium perfringens Toxin
4	Clostridium perfringens Toxins Type B, C, D and E
5	Cholera Toxins
6	Endotoxin of Shigella dysenteriae
7	Protein Toxins from Bordetella pertussis
8	Salmonella typhimurium and E. coli Neurotoxins
9	Toxins of Proteus mirabilis
10	Listeria monocytogenes Toxin

MICROBIAL TOXINS - VOL. IIB (BACTERIAL PROTEIN TOXINS) -
Edited by S. Kadis, T. C. Montie and S. J. Ajl. (In
Preparation). Academic Press, N. Y.

Diphtheria Toxin

MICROBIAL TOXINS - VOL. III (BACTERIAL PROTEIN TOXINS) -
Edited by T. C. Montie, S. Kadis and S. J. Ajl.
Academic Press, N. Y.

Chapter	Contents
1	Nature and Synthesis of Murine Toxins of Pasteurella pestis

MICROBIAL TOXINS - VOL. IV (BACTERIAL ENDOTOXINS) - Edited
by G. Weinbaum, S. Kadis and S. J. Ajl. Academic Press,
N. Y.

MICROBIAL TOXINS - VOL. V (BACTERIAL ENDOTOXINS) - Edited
by S. Kadis, G. Weinbaum and S. J. Ajl. Academic Press,
N. Y.

MICROBIAL TOXINS - VOL. VI (FUNGAL TOXINS) - Edited by
A. Ciegler, S. Kadis and S. Ajl. 1971. Academic Press,
N. Y. (563 pp.)

SECTION A - Aspergillus Toxins

SECTION B - Penicillin Toxins

MICROBIAL TOXINS - VOL. VII (ALGAL AND FUNGAL TOXINS) -
Edited by S. Kadis, A. Ciegler and S. Ajl. 1971. Academic Press, N. Y. (401 pp.)

SECTION A - Algal Toxins

SECTION B - Fungal Toxins, Toxins of Fusarium

MICROBIAL TOXINS - VOL. VIII (FUNGAL TOXINS) - Edited by
S. Kadis, A. Ciegler and S. Ajl. 1972. Academic Press, N. Y. (400 pp.)

SECTION A

MICROBIAL TRANSFORMATION OF STEROIDS AND ALKALOIDS -
H. Iizuka and A. Naito. 1967. University of Tokyo Press
(Tokyo) and University Park Press (State College, Penn.)
(294 pp.)

Contents   <u>Page</u>

<u>MICROBIOLOGICAL METHODS</u> - C. H. Collins. 1967. 2nd Edi-
tion, Plenum Press, N. Y.

<u>Part</u>   Contents   <u>Page</u>

<u>MICROBIOLOGY OF FOOD FERMENTATIONS</u> - C. S. Pederson. 1971.
AVI Publishing Company, Inc., Westport, Conn.

Chapter   Contents   <u>Page</u>

MINIATURIZED MICROBIOLOGICAL METHODS - Paul A. Hartman.
1968. Supplement 1 to Advances in Applied Microbiology.
Academic Press, N. Y. (227 pp.)

PFIZER HANDBOOK OF MICROBIAL METABOLITES, THE - Max Miller.
1961. Charles Pfizer & Co., McGraw Hill, N. Y. (772 pp.)

PRINCIPLES OF INDUSTRIAL MICROBIOLOGY - Alan Rhodes and Derek L. Fletcher. 1966. Pergamon Press, Oxford.

PROGRESS IN MICROBIOLOGICAL TECHNIQUES - Edited by C. H. Collins. 1967. Plenum Press, N. Y. (231 pp.)

RUMEN AND ITS MICROBES, THE - R. E. Hungate. 1966.
Academic Press, N. Y.

SAFETY IN MICROBIOLOGY - Editor D. A. Shapton and R. G.
Board. 1972. Society for Applied Bacteriology Technical
Series #6. Academic Press, N. Y. (266 pp.)

SINGLE CELL PROTEIN - Edited by Richard I. Mateles and
Steven R. Tannenbaum. 1968. MIT Press. (480 pp.)

TECHNIQUES IN EXPERIMENTAL VIROLOGY - Edited by R. J. C.
Harris. 1964. Academic Press, N. Y. (450 pp.)

THEORETICAL AND METHODOLOGICAL BASIS OF CONTINUOUS CULTURE
OF MICROORGANISMS - Edited by I. Malek and Z. Fencl.
1966. Academic Press, N. Y. (655 pp.)

TYPE REACTIONS IN FERMENTATION CHEMISTRY - L. L. Wallen,
F. H. Stodala and R. W. Jackson. 1959. Agricultural
Research Service, U. S. Dept. of Agriculture. (496 pp.)

YEASTS, THE - VOL. 1 (BIOLOGY OF YEASTS) - Edited by A. H.
Rose and J. S. Harrison. 1969. Academic Press, N. Y.

YEASTS, THE - VOL. 2 (PHYSIOLOGY AND BIOCHEMISTRY OF YEASTS) - Edited by A. H. Rose and J. S. Harrison. 1971. Academic Press, N. Y.

YEASTS, THE - VOL. 3 (YEAST TECHNOLOGY) - Edited by A. H. Rose and J. S. Harrison. 1970. Academic Press, N. Y.

SECTION II - A KEY TO THE REVIEW
LITERATURE IN INDUSTRIAL MICROBIOLOGY

The review articles included in the key are arranged chronologically under the following 57 broad subject headings:

49

The title of each review article cited in the guide is followed by a reference code. An example is decifered below:

Rheological Properties of Fermentation
Broths (2-1960) (265) A

Volume 2   Article begins   Advances in Applied
  1960   on pp. 265   Microbiology

All review articles included in this key have been taken from one of the following sources:

Code Letter

(A)   Advances in Applied Microbiology
        Academic Press, N. Y.

        Vol. 1, 1960 - Vol. 9, 1967 - Edited by W. W.
        Umbreit

        Vol. 10, 1968 - Vol. 12, 1970 - Edited by
        D. Perlman and W. W. Umbreit

        Vol. 13, 1970 - Vol. 15, 1972 - Edited by
        D. Perlman

        (Total 15 Volumes)

(B)   Bacteriological Reviews
        American Society for Microbiology, Washington,
        D. C.

        Vol. 24, 1960 - Vol. 37 (Parts 1 & 2), 1973

        (Total 13 1/2 Volumes)

(C)   Progress in Industrial Microbiology

        Vol. 1, 1959 - Vol. 4, 1964 - Heywood &
        Company Ltd., London

        Vol. 5, 1964 - Gordon & Breach, Science Pub-
        lisher, Great Britain

        Vol. 6, 1967 - Vol. 9, 1971 - CRC Press,
        Cleveland, Ohio

        (Total 9 Volumes)

Code Letter

(D)   Process Biochemistry
            Morgan-Grampian Ltd., London

            Vol. 1, 1966 - Vol. 8 (Issues 1 - 6), 1973

            (Total 7 1/2 Volumes)

(E)   Advances in Microbial Physiology
            Academic Press, N. Y.

            Vol. 1, 1967 - Vol. 7, 1972 - Edited by
              A. H. Rose and J. F. Wilkinson

            Vol. 8, 1972 - Vol. 9, 1973 - Edited by
              A. H. Rose and D. W. Tempest

            (Total 9 Volumes)

(F)   Developments in Industrial Microbiology

            Vol. 1, 1960 - Vol. 9, 1968 - Plenum Press,
              N. Y.

            Vol. 10, 1969 - Vol. 13, 1972 - Garamond/
              Pridemark Press, Baltimore, Md.

            Vol. 14, 1973 - Hennage Creative Printers,
              Washington, D. C.

            Contains the proceedings for each of the
            Annual Meetings of the Society for Industrial
            Microbiology.

            The Key contains the titles of each symposium
            consisting of several papers on the subject.
            The "Contributed Papers" are not, however, in-
            cluded in the Key.

            (Total 14 Volumes)

Code Letter

(G)   Advances in Drug Research
               Academic Press, N. Y.

               Vol. 1, 1964 - Vol. 6, 1972

               Key contains only those review articles that
               pertain to industrial microbiology.

               (Total 6 Volumes)

(H)   Annual Review of Microbiology
               Annual Reviews, Palo Alto, Calif.

               Edited by E. Clifton, S. Raffel and M. Starr

               Vol. 14, 1960 - Vol. 26, 1972

               (Total 13 Volumes)

(I)   Antimicrobial Agents and Chemotherapy

               Proceedings of the Interscience Conference on
               Antimicrobial Agents and Chemotherapy and pub-
               lished by the American Society for Microbio-
               logy, Bethesda, Md.

               Vol. 1, 1961 - Vol. 9, 1969

               Vol. 10, 1970 (Last volume published in this
                  format)

               Starting in 1971 the American Society for
               Microbiology began publishing a monthly jour-
               nal by the same name. As these articles are
               specific in nature, their titles are no
               longer included in this Key.

               (10 Volumes)

Code Letter

(J)   Advances in Biochemical Engineering
             Springer-Verlag, N. Y.

             Edited by T. K. Ghose

             Vol. 1, 1971

             (1 Volume)

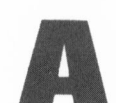

AGITATION/AERATION COMPLEX

Rheological Properties of Fermentation Broths
    (2-1960) (265) A

Fluid Mixing in Fermentation Processes
    (2-1960) (275) A

Scale-Up of Submerged Fermentations
    (2-1960) (289) A

Fermentation Kinetics and Model Processes
    (2-1960) (321) A

Studies in Aeration and Agitation
    (3-1961) (141) C

Aeration in the Laboratory
    (5-1963) (157) A

Compressors
    (1-1966) (291) D

Aeration and Agitation
    (1-1966) (307) D

Non-Newtonian and Biochemical Media
(1-1966) (435) D

Sulphite for Assessing Fermentor Performance
(2-1967) (57) D #5

Impellor-Power Consumption in Gas/Liquid Contactors
(2-1967) (27) D #8

Developments in Agitation and Aeration of Fermentation Systems
(8-1968) (1) C

Dissolved O_2 Measurement in Continuous Aseptic
Fermentations
(3-1968) (23) D #2

Dissolved O_2 Control
(4-1969) (27) D #3

Energy Costs of O_2 Transfer
(4-1969) (17) D #6

O_2 and Microbial Metabolism
(4-1969) (19) D #6

Mixing - Biochemical Industries
(4-1969) (25) D #6

Fluid Mixing
(4-1969) (51) D #8

Oxygen Metabolism by Microorganisms
(3-1969) (197) E

Effects of Impurities on O_2 Transfer
(6-1971) (33) D #4

Effect of Hyperbaric Oxygen on Microorganisms
(25-1971) (111) H

Modeling of Growth Processes with Two Liquid Phases:
A Review of Drop Phenomena, Mixing and Growth
(15-1972) (367) A

The Nature of Fermentation Fluids
(1-1972) (1) J

AIR MICROBIOLOGY

Aerosol Samplers
(2-1960) (31) A

Protection Against Infection in the Microbiological Laboratory: Devices and Procedures
(3-1961) (131) A

Second International Conference on Aerobiology
(Airborne Infection)
(30-1966) (485) B

Osmogenic Air Pollution
(3-1968) (53) D #2

Filtered Laminar Airflow Technology
(11-1970) (47) E

ALGAE

Biological Transformation of Solar Energy
(2-1960) (223) A

Phytoplankton and Marine Primary Production
(19-1965) (127) H

Industrial Uses of Algae
(3-1968) (11) D #10

Ecology, Physiology and Biochemistry of Blue-
Green Algae
(22-1968) (47) H

Biology and Physiology of the Coccolithophorids
(22-1968) (71) H

The Fine Structure of Blue-Green Algae
(22-1968) (15) H

Algae for Food and Feed
(4-1969) (45) D #6

Thermophilic Blue-Green Algae and the Thermal
Environment
(33-1969) (476) B

Processing Seaweed for Agar
(6-1971) (51) D #3

Physiology and Cytological Chemistry of Blue-
Green Algae
(37-1973) (32) B

AMINO ACIDS

The Production of Amino Acids by Fermentation
Processes
(1-1959) (201) A

Microbial Production of Amino Acids
(5-1964) (55) C

Amino-Acid Production
(1-1966) (359) D

Microbial Production of Amino Acids - Symposium
(7-1966) (3) F

Trends in Amino Acid Analyses
(4-1969) (37) D #8

ANATOMY (MICROBIAL)

The Anatomy of the Bacterial Surface
   (25-1961) (77) B

Fine Structure of Protozoa
   (15-1961) (47) H

Structure of Viruses
   (15-1961) (219) H

Structure of Some Animal Viruses and Significance
of Their Components
   (27-1963) (1) B

Cell Walls of Yeasts
   (17-1963) (15) H

Symposium on the Fine Structure and Replication
of Bacteria and Their Parts
   (29-1965) (277) B

Structure and Function in Protozoa
   (20-1966) (131) H

Developmental Changes During Formation and Breaking
of the Dormant State of Bacteria
   (20-1966) (169) H

Structure and Function of Bacterial Cell Membranes
   (21-1967) (417) H

Association of the Nucleus and the Membrane of Bacteria: A Morphological Study
   (32-1968) (39) B

The Fine Structure of Blue-Green Algae
   (22-1968) (15) H

Comparative Ultrastructure of Selected Aerobic
Spore-Forming Bacteria: A Freeze-Etching
Study
   (33-1969) (346) B

Cryo-Ultramicrotomy
(4-1969) (35) D #10

The Topography of the Bacterial Cell Wall
(23-1969) (159) H

Bacterial Flagella
(6-1971) (219) E

Walls and Membranes in Bacteria
(7-1972) (2) E

ANALYSES (CHEMICAL AND BIOCHEMICAL)

Methods for the Determination of Organic Acids
(3-1961) (343) A

Fusel Oil
(5-1963) (317) A

Gas Liquid Chromatography
(1-1966) (417) D

Chromatography Applications - Oil in Effluents
(2-1967) (33) D #5

Chromatography Applications - Meat
(2-1967) (29) D #5

Chromatography Applications - Steroids
(2-1967) (27) D #5

Chromatography Applications - Fish Products
(2-1967) (37) D #5

Chromatography Applications - Cheese
(2-1967) (35) D #5

Chromatography Applications - Packaged Meats
(2-1967) (30) D #5

Chromatography Applications - Food and Cereals
(2-1967) (21) D #5

Chromatography Applications - Wine
(2-1967) (34) D #5

A Continuous Flow Recording Respirometer
(2-1967) (21) D #10

Atomic Absorption Spectroscopy in the Biochemical
Industries
(2-1967) (27) D #6

Particle Size Analyses
(2-1967) (57) D #9

Determination of Chemical Structure
(2-1967) (13) D #5

Radiochromatography
(2-1967) (16) D #5

Chromatography Application
(3-1968) (21) D #3

Chromatography Applications - Pesticides
(3-1968) (21) D #3

Chromatography Applications - Water Pollution
(3-1968) (24) D #3

Chromatography Applications - Penicillin R & D
(3-1968) (31) D #3

Chromatography Applications - GC - IR Micro-
analysis
(3-1968) (34) D #3

Liquid Chromatography
(4-1969) (23) D #3

Automated Enzyme Assays
(4-1969) (57) D #3

Automated Biochemical Analysers
(4-1969) (67) D #3

Microcolorimetry
    (4-1969) (63) D #3

pH Electrodes in Fermentation
    (4-1969) (33) D #8

Trends in Amino Acid Analysis
    (4-1969) (37) D #8

Immuno-Electrophoresis
    (4-1969) (38) D #8

Spectrophotometry and Colorimetry - Product Survey
    (5-1970) (37) D #3

Spectroscopic Technique for the Study of Drug
    Interaction with Biological Systems
    (5-1970) (55) G

Atomic Absorption Spectrophotometry
    (5-1970) (35) D #1

Automated Analysis - Food and Allied Industries
    (5-1970) (29) D #3

The "Biological" Spectrophotometer
    (6-1971) (15) D #3

Computing in Biochemistry
    (6-1971) (19) D #3

Food Analysis by Gas Chromatography
    (7-1972) (13) D #2

Electroanalytical Techniques
    (7-1972) (23) D #2

Automation in Pharmaceutical Analyses
    (7-1972) (27) D #2

Analysis of the Government Chemist
    (7-1972) (37) D #2

A Nitrogen Detection Technique
    (7-1972) (41) D #2

Computor Control of a Gas Chromatograph
    (7-1972) (24) D #10

Principles and Practice of Hansch Analysis: A
Guide to Structure Activity Correlation for
the Medicinal Chemist
    (6-1972) (1) G

Mass Spectrometry in Drug Research
    (6-1972) (157) G

Views on Quality Control in the Pharmaceutical
Industry
    (8-1973) (11) D #2

Trace Analysis by Enzyme Inhibition and Activa-
tion
    (8-1973) (22) D #3

Automated and Instrumental Methods in Microbiology
    (14-1973) (67) F

ANIMAL HEALTH AND NUTRITION

The Arthropod-Born Viruses of Man and Other
Animals
    (14-1960) (261) H

Microbial Ecology of the Rumen
    (24-1960) (353) B

The Family Brucellaceae in Veterinary Research
    (15-1961) (93) H

Applied Microbiology in Animal Nutrition
    (4-1962) (77) A

Antimicrobials in Veterinary Medicine
    (3-1963) (588) I

The Rumen Bacteria and Protozoa
    (18-1964) (131) H

Viral Infections of Domestic Animals
    (18-1964) (269) H̲

E. coli and Neonatal Disease of Calves
    (29-1965) (75) B̲

Practical Aspects of Mycoplasmosis of Man and
    Animals
    (8-1967) (35) F̲

Foot and Mouth Disease
    (22-1968) (201) H̲

Microbiology of Grass Silage
    (3-1968) (27) D̲ #2

Rumen Microorganisms
    (4-1969) (53) D̲ #11

Mechanism of Perpetuation of Animal Viruses in
    Nature
    (33-1969) (404) B̲

Emerging Disease of Man and Animals
    (25-1971) (465) H̲

The Genus Erwinia: Enterobacteria Pathogenic to
    Plants and Animals
    (26-1972) (389) H̲

ANTIBIOTICS

Mechanism of Penicillin Biosynthesis
    (1-1959) (23) A̲

Status of Antibiotics in Plant Disease Control
    (1-1959) (87) A̲

The Influence of Medium Constituents on the Bio-
    synthesis of Penicillin
    (1-1959) (1) C̲

The Fermentation of the Tetracyclines
(1-1959) (45) C

Status of Antibiotics in Plant Disease Control
(1-1959) (87) A

The Biochemistry of Streptomycin Production
(2-1960) (131) C

Intermediary Metabolism and Antibiotic Synthesis
(3-1961) (293) A

Chloramphenicol
(25-1961) (32) B

Novobiocin
(3-1961) (91) C

The Assessment of the Interaction Between Antibacterial Drugs
(3-1961) (173) C

The Erythromycin Fermentation
(3-1961) (211) C

Nonmedical Aspects of Antibiotics
(2-1961) (105) F

Mode of Action: Biogenesis
(1-1961) (205) I

Clinical Evaluation of New Antibiotics - I
(1-1961) (286) I

Clinical Evaluation of New Antibiotics - II
(1-1961) (352) I

New Antibiotics
(1-1961) (436) I

New Penicillins: Chemistry and Biological Properties
(1-1961) (531) I

New Penicillins - I
(1-1961) (636) I

New Penicillins - II
(1-1961) (713) I

Synthetic Antimicrobials
(1-1961) (795) I

General
(1-1961) (892) I

The Classification of Actinomycetes in Relation to
Their Antibiotic Activity
(3-1961) (257) A

Chemistry of Antibiotics
(2-1962) (179) I

Synthetic Antimicrobials
(1-1962) (226) I

New Antibiotics
(2-1962) (543) I

Antibiotics - General
(2-1962) (619) I

Cephalosporins
(2-1962) (682) I

Antibiotics - In Vitro Activity
(2-1962) (787) I

The Actinomycetes and Their Antibiotics
(5-1963) (235) A

Infective Heredity of Multiple Drug Resistance
in Bacteria
(27-1963) (87) B

New Antibiotics
(3-1963) (1) I

Gentamicin - Lincomycin
(3-1963) (138) I

Oxacillins
(3-1963) (220) I

Cephalosporin - Penicillin - Nafcillin - Ampicillin
(3-1963) (243) I

Chemistry of Antibiotics
(3-1963) (346) I

Mode of Action of Antibiotics
(3-1963) (366) I

Antimicrobials - General
(3-1963) (402) I

Synthetic Microbials
(3-1963) (530) I

Side Reaction Attributed to Antimicrobial Agents
(3-1963) (785) I

Antibiotics in Control of Plant Disease
(17-1963) (243) H

Nonmedical Uses of Antibiotics
(6-1964) (91) A

Chloramphenicol
(4-1964) (137) C

Griseofulvin: Production and Biosynthesis
(4-1964) (165) C

Bacitracin, Its Manufacture and Uses
(5-1964) (93) C

Penicillins and Related Structures
(1-1964) G

New Antibiotics
(4-1964) (7) I

Antibiotics - General
(4-1964) (135) I

Penicillin and Cephalosporin
(4-1964) (188) I

Symposium on Penicillins and Cephalosporins
   (4-1964) (274) I

In Vitro Studies
   (4-1964) (311) I

Mode of Action
   (4-1964) (474) I

Synthetic Antimicrobials
   (4-1964) (545) I

Symposium on Synthetic Antimicrobials
   (4-1964) (619) I

The Bacteriocins
   (29-1965) (25) B

Antibiotics and Their Mechanisms
   (19-1965) (209) H

25 Years of Penicillin Therapy in Perspective
   (5-1965) (1) I

A Quarter Century of the Antibiotic Era
   (5-1965) (9) I

Chemistry of Antibiotics and Other Antimicrobial
   Agents and the Biosynthesis of Antibiotics
   (5-1965) (115) I

Pharmacology and Pharmacokinetics of the Antimicrobial Agent
   (5-1965) (168) I

Experimental Studies and the Mode of Action of
   Antimicrobial Agents
   (5-1965) (256) I

Clinical Studies of Antimicrobial Agents
   (5-1965) (610) I

New Antimicrobial Agents
   (5-1965) (734) I

Symposium on the Chemistry of Antibiotics
(5-1965) (951) <u>I</u>

Symposium on Biogenesis of Antibiotics
(5-1965) (982) <u>I</u>

Symposium on Clinically Important Antibiotics as
Biochemical Tools
(5-1965) (992) <u>I</u>

Symposium on the Penetration of Drugs into Tissue
(5-1965) (1016) <u>I</u>

Symposium on Chemotherapy of Mycobacterial Diseases
(5-1965) (1058) <u>I</u>

Are New Antibiotics Needed?
(5-1965) (1107) <u>I</u>

Round Table on Chemotherapy of Venereal Diseases
(5-1965) (1115) <u>I</u>

Round Table on Antifungal Agents
(5-1965) (1120) <u>I</u>

Microbial Ecology and Applied Microbiology
(8-1966) (61) <u>A</u>

Microbial Synthesis of Penicillins, Part 1
(1-1966) (334) <u>D</u>

Microbial Synthesis of Penicillins, Part 2
(1-1966) (373) <u>D</u>

Mechanisms by which Antibiotics Increase the Incidence
and Severity of Candiasis and Alter the Immunological Defenses
(30-1966) (442) <u>B</u>

Resistance of Plants to Infectious Agents
(20-1966) (337) <u>H</u>

Clinical Evaluation of Antimicrobial Agents in
Humans
(6-1966) (42) <u>I</u>

Genetic Aspects of Drug Resistance
 (6-1966) (212) I

Symposium: Epidemiology of Drug Resistant
 Infections
 (6-1966) (245) I

Mycoplasma, Protoplasts and Antibiotic Action
 (6-1966) (297) I

Enzymatic Inhibition of Antibiotic Action
 (6-1966) (316) I

In Vitro and In Vivo Action of Antimicrobial
 Agents
 (6-1966) (352) I

Production and Biological and Chemical Properties
 of Antimicrobial Agents and Their Derivatives
 (6-1966) (563) I

Symposium: Identification Aspects of the Production and Metabolism of Antibiotics
 (6-1966) (637) I

Symposium: Chemical Modification of Antibiotics
 (6-1966) (670) I

Symposium: Nonpharmaceutical Use of Antibiotics
 (6-1966) (737) I

Cephalosporins
 (4-1967) G

Production of Polyene Antifungal Agents by Streptomycetes
 (6-1967) (1) C

Production of Rifamycins
 (6-1967) (21) C

Studies on the Mechanism of Actinomycin Biosynthesis
 (6-1967) (61) C

Antibiotics - A Review
   (3-1968) (45) D #10

Antibiotics in the Control of Plant Pathogens
   (10-1968) (313) A

Early Days of Antimicrobial Therapy
   (8-1968) (1) I

Drug Resistance and Mechanism of Action of Antimicrobial Agents
   (8-1968) (7) I

Chemical Studies on Antimicrobial Agents and
  Semisynthetic Antibiotics
   (8-1968) (229) I

New Antimicrobial Agents
   (8-1968) (229) I

Evaluation of Antimicrobial Agents in Humans
   (8-1968) (274) I

In Vitro Antimicrobial Action
   (8-1968) (382) I

In Vivo Antimicrobial Action and Experimental
  Studies in Animals
   (8-1968) (474) I

Fusidane Type Antibiotics
   (4-1969) (11) D #12

Successes and Failures in the Search for Antibiotics
   (11-1969) (1) A

Structure - Activity Relationships of Semisynthetic Penicillins
   (11-1969) (17) A

Resistance to Antimicrobial Agents
   (11-1969) (77) A

Antibiotics as Probes to Elucidate Cell Biochemistry
   (9-1969) (5) I

Pharmacological Action of Antimicrobial Agents
(9-1969) (35) I

Mechanism of Action and Antimicrobial Resistance
(9-1969) (56) I

Chemical Studies on Antimicrobial Agents and Semisynthetic Antibiotics
(9-1969) (111) I

New Antibiotics and Antimicrobial Agents
(9-1969) (200) I

Studies of Phosphonomycin
(9-1969) (284) I

In Vitro Antimicrobial Action and Experimental
Studies in Animals
(9-1969) (445) I

Sporulation and the Production of Antibiotics,
Exoenzymes and Exotoxins
(33-1969) (48) B

Biochemistry and Regulation of Streptomycin and
Mannosidostreptomycinase Formation
(34-1970) (1) B

Occurrence, Chemistry and Toxicology of Microbial
Peptide - Lactones
(12-1970) (189) A

Rifamycin Antibiotics - Initial Development
(5-1970) (31) D #11

Antibiotic Effects of Sea Water
(5-1970) (39) D #11

Structure - Activity Relationships Among Semisynthetic Cephalosporins
(13-1970) (163) A

Structure - Activity Relationships Among Tetra-
cycline Series
(13-1970) (237) A

Antimicrobial Agents and Membrane Function
   (4-1970) (46) E

Synthetic Antimicrobial Agents and Chemical
   Studies
   (10-1970) I

New Penicillins
   (10-1970) I

Pharmacological Studies and Toxicology of Antimicrobial Agents
   (10-1970) I

Antimicrobial Resistance and Mechanisms of Action
   (10-1970) I

In Vitro Antimicrobial Action
   (10-1970) I

Microbial Transformation of Antibiotics
   (6-1971) (13) D #7

Actions of the Rifamycins
   (35-1971) (290) B

Prevalence and Distribution of Antibiotic Producing Actinomycetes
   (14-1971) (73) A

Microbial Transformations of Antibiotics
   (14-1971) (123) A

In Vivo Evaluation of Antibacterial Chemothera-
   peutic Substances
   (14-1971) (151) A

Modification of Lincomycin
   (14-1971) (185) A

Structure - Activity Relationships in Coumermycins
   (15-1972) (231) A

Chloramphenicol
   (15-1972) (297) A

Rifampin: A Semisynthetic Derivative of Rifamycin
- A Prototype for the Future
(26-1972) (85) H̲

Rifamycins: A General Review
(26-1972) (199) H̲

Chemistry and Biology of the Polyene Macrolide Antibiotics
(37-1973) (166) B̲

APPLIED MICROBIOLOGY

Training for Careers in Microbiology
(1-1960) (3) F̲

Industrial Fermentations
(14-1960) (99) H̲

Microbiology and the Microbiologist
(27-1963) (243) B̲

Global Impacts of Applied Microbiology: An
Appraisal
(6-1964) (2) A̲

A Discussion of the Training of Applied Microbiologists
(6-1964) (227) A̲

Microbial Dissonance
(29-1965) (269) B̲

Symposium on Information Science
(29-1965) (505) B̲

National Science and Microbiology
(31-1967) (3) B̲

And Gladly Wolde He Lerne and Gladly Teche
(31-1967) (175) B̲

The Education of a Microbiologist; Some Reflections
    (21-1967) (1) H

Who Speaks for Microbiology
    (33-1969) (363) B

Training for the Biochemical Industries
    (11-1969) (283) A

Contributions Toward the Development of General
  Microbiology
    (24-1970) (1) H

Development of the Fermentation Industries in
  Great Britain
    (14-1971) (1) A

Microbial Criteria of Environment Qualities
    (25-1971) (563) H

Training a Microbiologist
    (26-1972) (1) H

ASSAYS (MICROBIOLOGICAL)

A Commentary on Microbiological Assaying
    (2-1950) (65) A

Microbiological Assay
    (1-1959) (93) C

The Gram Stain and the Etiology of Lobar Pneumonia,
  An Historical Note
    (24-1960) (261) B

Assay Methodology in the Fermentation Industry
    (2-1961) (157) F

International Integration of Antibiotic Sensitivity
  Tests
    (2-1962) (867) I

Rapid Microbiological Determinations with Radio-
isotopes
(5-1963) (95) A

Bacteriophage Typing of Staphylococci
(27-1963) (253) B

Some Recent Advances in Diagnostic Medical Bacteriology
(17-1963) (565) H

Media and Methods for Isolation and Enumeration
of the Enterococci
(8-1966) (253) A

Low Level Microbiological Assays
(10-1969) (3) F

Bacterial Cell Counts
(5-1970) (35) D #3

Automated Bioassay of Antibiotics using Direct
Turbidimetry
(6-1971) (25) D #3

Drop Method for Microbial Counts
(6-1971) (31) D #5

Some Aspects of Cosmetic Microbiology
(12-1971) (155) F

Correlative Microbiological Assays
(15-1972) (147) A

Automated and Instrumental Methods in Microbiology
(14-1973) (67) F

B

BREWERY OPERATIONS

Microbial Control Methods in the Brewery
(2-1960) (113) A

Microbiological Aspects of Brewing
(4-1963) (153) F

Biochemistry of Malting
(1-1966) (55) D

What's Involved in Beer Storage
(1-1966) (113) D

Tower Fermentation of Beer
(1-1966) (215) D

Biochemistry of Mashing
(1-1966) (241) D

Amino Acids in Malting and Brewing
(1-1966) (412) D

Brewing Behaviour of Hops
(2-1967) (31) D #2

Continuous Food Processes
(3-1968) (58) D #9

Modern Brewing in (1) Britain (2) Germany (3)
Finland
(4-1969) (23, 27, 29) D #5

EBC and International Brewing
(4-1969) (21) D #5

Brewing Beer with Enzymes
(4-1969) (33) D #5

Candle Filter in Brewing
(4-1969) (66) D #5

Advances in Brewing Separation
(4-1969) (37) D #9

Technology of Brewing Carbohydrates
(5-1970) (39) D #2

Pure Yeast Cultures in Brewing
(5-1970) (15) D #4

Malt Extracts
(5-1970) (19) D #4

Economics of Brewery Fermentation
(5-1970) (25) D #4

A Practical Assessment of Hop Extracts
(5-1970) (33) D #4

Glucoamylases in Modern Brewing
(5-1970) (37) D #4

Cleaning and Sterilizing in Brewing
(5-1970) (41) D #4

Isomerized Hop Extracts
(5-1970) (49) D #4

Microbial Enzymes for Beer
(5-1970) (60) D #4

Technology of Barley Brewing
(5-1970) (46) D #8

Spoilage Organisms in Breweries
(6-1971) (15) D #4

Centrifuges and Spent Grain Problems
(6-1971) (37) D #4

Enzyme Activity in Germinating Barley
(6-1971) (19) D #4

Carbohydrate Balance and Its Economics in Brewing
(6-1971) (28) D #7

Carbohydrate Composition of Malt
(6-1971) (32) D #7

Microbiology of Brewing
(25-1971) (583) H

Design of Modern Malting
(7-1972) (17) D #4

Amino Acid Composition of Malt
(7-1972) (26) D #4

Control of Beer Foam
(7-1972) (29) D #4

Preservation of Beer
(7-1972) (32) D #4

Views on Quality Control in the Brewery
(8-1973) (14) D #2

Glycerol and Organic Acids of Malt
(8-1973) (22) D #4

Scale Treatment in a Brewery
(8-1973) (25) D #4

C

CANCER CHEMOTHERAPY

Antitumor Antibiotics
  (1-1960) (79) F

Screening for and Biological Characteristics of
  Antitumor Agents Using Microorganisms
  (3-1961) (223) A

Cancer Chemotherapy
  (1-1961) (148) I

Cancer Chemotherapy
  (2-1962) (731) I

Some Aspects of the Problem of Immunity Against
  Transplanted and Spontaneous Tumors
  (26-1962) (336) B

Viral Leukemias in Mice
  (16-1962) (75) H

Response of Cell and Organism to Infection with
  Avian Tumor Viruses
  (26-1962) (1) B

Microorganisms and the Molecular Biology of Cancer
   (5-1963) (65) <u>A</u>

Malignant Transformation by Polyoma Virus
   (17-1963) (167) <u>H</u>

Symposium on Antineoplastic Antibiotics
   (4-1964) (500) <u>I</u>

Chemotherapy of Cancer and Viral Infections
   (5-1965) (481) <u>I</u>

Symposium on Cancer Chemotherapy
   (5-1965) (1079) <u>I</u>

Development and Evaluation of Antiviral and Antitumor Agents
   (6-1966) (483) <u>I</u>

Tumor Antigens
   (20-1966) (223) <u>H</u>

Virus Leukemia in the Mouse
   (21-1967) (529) <u>H</u>

Microbial Models of Tumor Metabolism
   (9-1967) (69) <u>A</u>

Virus Leukemia in the Mouse
   (21-1967) (529) <u>H</u>

The Oncogenic DNA Viruses: A Review of In Vitro
   Transformation Studies
   (22-1968) (391) <u>H</u>

Occurrence, Chemistry and Toxicology of Microbial
   Peptides - Lactones
   (12-1970) (189) <u>A</u>

Rifamycin Antibiotics - Initial Development
   (5-1970) (31) <u>D</u> #11

Mechanism of Cell Transformation by RNA Tumor
   Viruses
   (25-1971) (609) <u>H</u>

Carcinogens Produced by Fungi
(26-1972) (279) H

CONTINUOUS FERMENTATIONS

Continuous Industrial Fermentations
(1-1959) (215) A

Continuous Culture of Microorganisms
(15-1961) (27) H

Biological Aspects of Continuous Cultivation of
Microorganisms
(4-1962) (101) A

Continuous Culture: Theory and Applications
(1-1966) (77) D

Continuous Lactic Fermentation
(1-1966) (441) D

Tower Fermentation of Beer
(1-1966) (215) D

Continuous Culture
(6-1967) (209) C

Continuous Cultivation of Microorganisms
(3-1968) (41) D #1

Microbial Interactions in Continuous Culture
(10-1968) (269) A

Dissolved Oxygen Measurement in Continuous Aseptic
Fermentations
(3-1968) (23) D #2

Industrial Applications of Continuous Culture:
Pharmaceutical Products and Other Products and
Processes
(13-1970) (399) A

Laboratory Scale Continuous Fermentor
(5-1970) (17) D #2

The Place of Continuous Culture in Microbiological
Research
(4-1970) (223) E

Continuous Culture - 1971
(7-1972) (21) D #7

Studies on Continuous Fermentation of Indian Cane
Sugar Molasses by Yeast
(8-1973) (23) D #2

CULTURE MAINTENANCE

Preservation of Bacteria by Lyophilization
(3-1961) (1) A

Stability and Degeneration of Microbial Cultures
on Repeated Transfer
(5-1963) (189) A

Selection, Improvement and Preservation of Microorganisms
(5-1964) (3) C

Preservation of Cultures
(4-1964) (189) C

Use and Abuse of Culture Collections
(1-1966) (339) D

D

DAIRY MICROBIOLOGY

The Lactobacilli - I
(2-1960) (1) C

The Importance of Bacterial Viruses in Industrial
Processes, Especially in the Dairy Industry
(4-1962) (51) A

The Lactobacilli - II
(4-1964) (95) C

Butter Manufacture
(1-1966) (207) D

Behavior of Microorganisms Associated with Dairy
Products - Symposium
(3-1968) (19) D #1

Ultra High Temperature Treatment of Milk
(1-1966) (103) D

Cheddar Cheese Manufacture - Part 1
(2-1967) (5) D #2

Cheddar Cheese Manufacture - Part 2
(2-1967) (23) D #3

Cheddar Cheese Manufacture - Part 3
(2-1967) (49) D #5

Cream Processing
(3-1968) (19) D #1

Blue Veined Cheese
(3-1968) (11) D #5

Biocides in Bulk Milk Tank Handling
(3-1968) (27) D #11

Dairy Fermentation Processes
(4-1969) (13) D #2

Ice Cream Refrigeration Equipment
(4-1969) (31) D #10

Recent Developments in Milk Products
(6-1971) (21) D #12

Cheesemaking - Enzymology or Bacteriology
(7-1972) (33) D #11

Mixer Emulsifiers in the Dairy Industry
(7-1972) (15) D #5

Cheese Manufacture - A Semicontinuous Process
(7-1972) (20) D #5

The Cheese Process - Microbiology and Enzymology
(7-1972) (33) D #6

Changing Technology in UK Dairying
(8-1973) (22) D #5

DETERIORATION (MICROBIAL)

Deterioration of Proteins
(1-1960) (121) F

Deterioration of Wood by Lower Fungi
(1-1960) (147) F

Deterioration of Materials
(2-1961) (45) F

Microbiology of Paint Films
(5-1963) (217) A

Microbial Aspects of Leather and Fabrics
(5-1964) (5) F

Microbial Deterioration of Resin Systems
(9-1968) (189) F

Microbial Corrosion
(3-1968) (17) D #12

DISTILLERY OPERATIONS

Gin Manufacture
(1-1966) (355) D

Distillery Byproduct Recovery
(1-1966) (407) D

Low Pressure Distillation #1
(2-1967) (25) D #1

Low Pressure Distillation #2
(2-1967) (37) D #3

Manufacture of Scotch Malt Whiskey
(3-1968) (9) D #1

Molecular Distillation
(3-1968) (23) $\underline{D}$ #5

Manufacture of German Gin
(3-1968) (28) $\underline{D}$ #10

Composition of Whiskey Flavor
(5-1970) (13) $\underline{D}$ #7

Irish Whiskey
(5-1970) (17) $\underline{D}$ #10

Manufacture of Brandy
(6-1971) (25) $\underline{D}$ #2

Rum Manufacture
(6-1971) (35) $\underline{D}$ #7

Views on Quality Control in Distilling
(8-1973) (18) $\underline{D}$ #2

E

ELECTRICAL GENERATION (MICROBIAL)

Generation of Electricity by Microbial Action
(5-1963) (51) A

Biochemical Fuel Cells
(4-1963) (51) F

Symposium on Bioelectrochemistry of Microorganisms
(30-1966) (67) B

Biochemical Fuel Cells
(9-1971) (1) C

ENZYMES

Enzyme Localization in Bacteria
(14-1960) (24) H

Symposium on Multiple Forms of Enzymes and Control
Mechanisms
(27-1963) (155) B

Enzymes and Their Applications
(6-1964) (207) A

Microbial Amylases
(7-1965) (273) A

Regulation on Enzyme Activity in Microorganisms
(19-1965) (105) H

Complementation at the Molecular Level of Enzyme
Interaction
(19-1965) (267) H

Fungal Amylase Production
(1-1966) (234) D

Enzymes in Industry
(1-1966) (279) D

Crystalline Oxygenases of Pseudomonads
(30-1966) (720) B

Penicillinacylase
(30-1966) (761) B

Enzyme Synthesis in Micro-organisms
(2-1967) (17) D #2

Recent Developments in the Production and Industrial Applications of Amylolytic Enzymes Derived
from Filamentous Fungi
(6-1967) (95) C

Large Scale Isolation of Enzymes
(2-1967) (13) D #7

Enzyme Extraction from Animal and Plant Tissues
(3-1968) (22) D #8

Manufacture of Pectinases (Part 1)
(3-1968) (27) D #8

Insolubilized Enzymes
(3-1968) (36) D #8

Use of Bacteriolytic Enzymes in Determination of
Wall Structure and Their Role in Cell Metabolism
(32-1968) (425) B

Production of Bacterial Amylases
(3-1968) (53) D #11

Proteins and Enzymes as Taxonomic Tools
(10-1968) (137) A

Sporulation and the Production of Antibiotics,
Exoenzymes and Exotoxins
(33-1969) (48) B

Enzymes in Washing Powders
(4-1969) (30) D #2

Biosyntheses of Bacterial Lysozomes
(4-1969) (53) D #4

Brewing Beer with Enzymes
(4-1969) (33) D #5

Enzymes for Breakage of Microorganisms
(4-1969) (63) D #5

New Sources of Rennet
(4-1969) (13) D #7

Proteolytic Enzymes
(4-1969) (19) D #8

Microbial Enzymes for Alcohol Production
(4-1969) (23) D #8

Manufacture of Pectinases
(4-1969) (27) D #8

Disruption of Mycelia for Enzymes
(4-1969) (19) D #12

Automated Enzyme Assays
 (4-1969) (57) <u>D</u> #3

Regulation of Enzyme Function
 (23-1969) (47) <u>H</u>

Plasmin and Fibrinolysis
 (5-1970) (46) <u>D</u> #2

Microbial Rennet - Mucor Miehi
 (5-1970) (34) <u>D</u> #4

Enzymes in Clinical Diagnosis
 (5-1970) (13) <u>D</u> #8

Water Insoluble Enzymes
 (5-1970) (14) <u>D</u> #8

Enzymatic De-Sizing of Textiles
 (5-1970) (17) <u>D</u> #8

UK Plant for Purified Enzymes
 (5-1970) (22) <u>D</u> #8

How Active are Commercial Enzymes
 (5-1970) (39) <u>D</u> #8

Enzymes - Laboratory Scale Production
 (5-1970) (62) <u>D</u> #9

The Evolution of Bacterial Enzyme Systems
 (24-1970) (429) <u>H</u>

Microbial Enzymes for Beer
 (5-1970) (60) <u>D</u> #4

Aliphatic Amidases in Pseudomonas aeruginosa
 (4-1970) (179) <u>E</u>

Glucoamylases in Modern Brewing
 (5-1970) (37) <u>D</u> #4

Enzyme Activity in Germinating Barley
 (6-1971) (19) <u>D</u> #4

Microbial Enzymes in Brewing
    (6-1971) (29) D̲ #4

Enzymes as Additives in Detergents
    (12-1971) (11) F̲

Enzyme Purification by Gel Filtration
    (6-1971) (39) D̲ #9

Microbial Proteases
    (6-1971) (17) D̲ #8

Enzymes in Clinical Biochemistry
    (6-1971) (23) D̲ #8

Microbial Intracellular Enzymes
    (6-1971) (27) D̲ #8

Biochemical Reactors
    (6-1971) (29) D̲ #8

Insolubilized Catalase
    (6-1971) (42) D̲ #8

Enzyme Reactors in Food Technology
    (6-1971) (11) D̲ #10

Synthesis of Enzymes During the Cell Cycle
    (6-1971) (47) E̲

Enzyme Activity in Germinating Barley
    (6-1971) (19) D̲ #4

α-Glucosidase and Leavening of Bakers Yeast
    (7-1972) (16) D̲ #5

Fibre Entrapped Enzymes
    (7-1972) (9) D̲ #8

Pectic Substances and Pectinolytic Enzymes
    (7-1972) (13) D̲ #8

Disappearing Enzymes
    (7-1972) (18) D̲ #8

Bacillus Derived Detergent Enzymes
(7-1972) (23) D #8

Externally Added Beta Glucanase
(7-1972) (27) D #8

Medical Applications of Microbial Enzymes
(15-1972) (1) A

Immobilized Enzymes
(15-1972) (13) A

Microbial Rennets
(15-1972) (39) A

A Simplified Kinetic Approach to Cellulose-
Cellulase System
(1-1972) (55) J

Production and Application of Enzymes
(1-1972) (77) J

Overproduction of Microbial Metabolites and
Enzymes Due to Alteration of Regulation
(1-1972) (113) J

Cellulase #2: Applications
(8-1973) (20) D #5

Cellulase #1: Sources and Technology
(8-1973) (35) D #4

Bacteria, Enzymes and Wood Permeability
(8-1973) (30) D #6

The β-Lactamases of Gram Negative Bacteria and
Their Possible Physiological Role
(9-1973) (89) E

EXTRACTION AND ISOLATION TECHNIQUES

Fermentation Metabolites: Part 1: Isolation on a
  Laboratory Scale
  (1-1966) (89) <u>D</u>

Fermentation Metabolites: Part 2: Isolation on
  Pilot Plant Scale
  (1-1966) (156) <u>D</u>

Extraction of Pectin
  (1-1966) (378) <u>D</u>

Gas-Liquid Chromatography
  (1-1966) (417) <u>D</u>

Fermentation Metabolites: Part 3: Less Common
  Unit Operations
  (1-1966) (431) <u>D</u>

Extraction of Fruit Juices
  (1-1966) (457) <u>D</u>

Low Pressure Distillation
  (2-1967) (25) <u>D</u> #1

Low Pressure Distillation - Part 2
  (2-1967) (37) <u>D</u> #3

Separation Techniques - Wine
  (2-1967) (32) <u>D</u> #9

Separation Techniques - Brewing
  (2-1967) (41) <u>D</u> #9

Separation Techniques - Vegetable Preparation
  (2-1967) (27) <u>D</u> #9

Separation Techniques - Sludge Dewatering
  (2-1967) (34) <u>D</u> #9

Separation Techniques - Vegetable Oil Refining
  (2-1967) (42) <u>D</u> #9

Separation Techniques - Fermentation Products
      (2-1967) (28) D #9

Separation Techniques - Water
      (2-1967) (29) D #9

Ion Exchange Celluloses for Biochemical Separations
      (2-1967) (7) D #8

Spray Dryers for Sterile Products
      (2-1967) (15) D #6

Breakage of Microorganisms
      (2-1967) (41) D #7

Large Scale Isolation of Enzymes
      (2-1967) (13) D #7

Clarification of Culture Fluids
      (3-1968) (19) D #9

Flocculation and Coagulation
      (3-1968) (17) D #10

Liquid Sprays
      (4-1969) (37) D #2

Recovery and Purification of Biochemicals
      (11-1969) (159) A

Collecting of Microbial Cells
      (12-1970) (121) A

Centrifuges in the Pharmaceutical Industry
      (5-1970) (32) D #9

Product Survey - Separation and Filtration
      (5-1970) (35) D #9

Ultrasonic Treatment for Microorganisms
      (6-1971) (22) D #3

Plasma Protein Fractionation
      (6-1971) (29) D #9

Recent Developments in Separation Methods
(6-1971) (35) D #9

Novel Shock Tube Cell Disruptor
(6-1971) (32) D #11

Protein and Fat Recovery from Effluents
(7-1972) (15) D #3

Continuous Extractor for Liquorice
(7-1972) (18) D #3

Fractionation of Blood by Centrifugation
(7-1972) (20) D #3

Foam Spray Drying Using a Centrifugal Atomiser
(7-1972) (25) D #3

Centrifuges for Animal By Products
(7-1972) (37) D #3

Reverse Osmosis in the Concentration of Food
(7-1972) (40) D #3

A Development in Reverse Osmosis
(7-1972) (25) D #6

Concentration of Microbial Cells
(13-1972) (159) F

Practice and Potential of Liquid Chromatography
(7-1972) (11) D #9

Reverse Osmosis of Milk and Whey
(7-1972) (17) D #9

Separation of Cells from Culture Media
(1-1972) (31) J

Industrial Applications of Gel Filtration - 1 Whey
(8-1973) (13) D #3

Developments of Hygienic Plant for Reverse Osmosis
and Ultrafiltration Applications
(8-1973) (18) D #3

F

FERMENTATION EQUIPMENT AND TECHNIQUES

Protected Fermentation
    (1-1959) (1) A

Control Applications in Fermentation
    (2-1960) (356) A

Uses of Ion Exchange Resins in Microbiology
    (24-1960) (251) B

Developments in Fermentor Design and Fermentation
    Control
    (2-1960) (103) C

Electrical Weighing in the Biochemistry Industries
    (1-1966) (37) D

Controlled Volume Pumps
    (1-1966) (58) D

Continuous Level Measurement
    (1-1966) (145) D

A Survey of Laboratory Fermentors
    (2-1967) (7) D #3

Media for Industrial Fermentations
    (2-1967) (19) D #6

Ampholytic Surface Active Agents
    (2-1967) (28) D #11

Antifoams
    (2-1967) (47) D #10

Discrete Level Detection
    (2-1967) (35) D #1

Stainless Steel in Biochemical Plants
    (2-1967) (19) D #7

Plastic Storage Tanks for Biochemical Liquids
    (2-1967) (36) D #10

Valves in the Biochemical Industries
    (2-1967) (31) D #4

Reinforced Plastics for Storage
    (2-1967) (27) D #7

The Package Pumping Station
    (2-1967) (51) D #51

Enrichment Culture
    (21-1967) (49) H

Preparative Scale Culture Vessels
    (3-1968) (15) D #3

Large-Scale Growth of Microorganisms and Their
    Products
    (3-1968) (51) D #4

Economics of Fermentor Design
    (3-1968) (28) D #5

Economics of Fermentor Operation - Part 2
    (3-1968) (56) D #6

A Survey of Pilot Fermentors
    (3-1968) (17) D #8

Culture of Higher Fungi
(8-1968) (73) <u>C</u>

Organization of Information About Microorganisms
(7-1968) (125) <u>C</u>

Fermentation Media
(4-1969) (17) <u>D</u> #1
a. Malt and Cereal Adjuncts
(17)
b. Yeast Products from Whey
(21)
c. Laboratory Cultures
(25)
d. Chemical Effluents
(29)
e. Sugar and Molasses
(34)

The Shaker in Bioengineering
(4-1969) (35) <u>D</u> #3

Computor Control of Batch Fermentation
(4-1969) (43) <u>D</u> #3

Dialysis Culture of Microorganisms: Design, Theory
and Results
(33-1969) (1) <u>B</u>

Shake Flask Cultivation of Bacteria
(5-1970) (7) <u>D</u> #2

Installation of Fermentation Pilot Plant
(5-1970) (10) <u>D</u> #2

Costs of Fermentor Instrumentation
(5-1970) (13) <u>D</u> #2

Laboratory Scale Continuous Fermentor
(5-1970) (17) <u>D</u> #2

Dosing Valve for Fermentors
(5-1970) (21) <u>D</u> #2

pH Sterilizable Probes
(5-1970) (25) <u>D</u> #3

Fermentor Design
      (12-1970) (153) <u>A</u>

Design of Fermentor Installations
      (5-1970) (51) <u>D</u> #8

Comparison of Surface Active Agents
      (5-1970) (19) <u>D</u> #11

Perforated Plate Column Fermentor
      (5-1970) (52) <u>D</u> #11

Mathematical Models for Fermentation Processes
      (13-1970) (419) <u>A</u>

Safety in the Microbiological Laboratory
      (5-1970) (27) <u>D</u> #6

Safety in Fermentation Processes
      (5-1970) (30) <u>D</u> #6

Metering Pumps
      (5-1970) (25) <u>D</u> #12

Technological Advances in Fermentation Equipment
      (6-1971) (15) <u>D</u> #2

"FERMT" - A Fermentation Process Game
      (6-1971) (38) <u>D</u> #2

Wood Hydrolysis and Fermentation
      (6-1971) (19) <u>D</u> #2

Foams and Antifoams in Fermentation
      (6-1971) (23) <u>D</u> #21

Survey of Laboratory Fermentors
      (6-1971) (36) <u>D</u> #8

Protection from Radioactive Chemicals
      (6-1971) (19) <u>D</u> #6

Fermentation Equipment
      (14-1971) (231) <u>A</u>

Ultrafiltration of Biological Materials
    (4-1969) (47) D #9

Filtration of Edible Oils
    (4-1969) (52) D #9

Pleated Membrane Cartridge
    (4-1969) (55) D #9

Product Survey - Separation and Filtration
    (4-1969) (59) D #9

Filtration in Food Processes
    (4-1969) (47) D #10

Overpressure Filter
    (4-1969) (66) D #5

Candle Filter in Brewing
    (4-1969) (66) D #5

Bacterial Filtration of Air
    (5-1970) (47) D #5

Filtration Through Deep Beds
    (6-1971) (21) D #9

High Volume Air Sterilization
    (6-1971) (25) D #9

Sheet Filters
    (6-1971) (53) D #9

Standardizing the Testing and Sizing of Filter Cakes
    (7-1972) (23) D #10

FOOD MICROBIOLOGY

Microbial Fat: Microorganisms as Potential Fat
    Producers
    (1-1959) (165) C

Preservation of Foods and Drugs by Ionizing
Radiations
(1-1959) (49) A

Fish Microbiology
(4-1964) (97) F

Potential for Increasing Food Production Through
Microbiology
(29-1965) (251) B

Microbiology of Freeze Dried Foods
(7-1965) (305) A

Podding and Vining of Peas and Beans
(1-1966) (171) D

Vacuum Concentration of Fruit Juices
(1-1966) (229) D

Advances in Breadmaking
(1-1966) (366) D

Extraction of Fruit Juices
(1-1966) (457) D

Microorganisms as Potential Food Sources
(7-1966) (203) F

Nisin and Food Preservation
(1-1966) (461) D

Radiation Sterilization of Meat
(1-1966) (487) D

Bacteriology of Fish Spoilage and Preservation
(6-1967) (169) C

Discoloration in Cooked Ham
(2-1967) (49) D #3

Separation Techniques - Vegetable Oil Refining
(2-1967) (42) D #9

Cider Manufacture
(2-1967) (37) D #11

Coffee Manufacture
    (2-1967) (15) D #10

Tea Manufacture
    (2-1967) (9) D #6

Storage of Fruit Juices
    (2-1967) (47) D #6

Curing of Pig Meat - Part 1
    (2-1967) (48) D #7

Curing of Pig Meat - Part 2
    (2-1967) (32) D #8

Curing of Pig Meat - Part 3
    (2-1967) (67) D #9

Biochemical Aspects of Breadmaking
    (2-1967) (18) D #4

Separation Techniques - Vegetable Preparation
    (2-1967) (27) D #9

Food Borne Salmonellosis
    (21-1967) (495) H

Air Blast Freezing of Fish
    (2-1967) (42) D #6

Storage of Grain
    (3-1968) (46) D #1

Biscuit Manufacture
    (3-1968) (58) D #3

Microorganisms in the Confectionary Industry
    (3-1968) (19) D #5

Protein Recovery from Fruit Juices
    (3-1968) (51) D #5

Clarification of Fruit Juices
    (3-1968) (38) D #5

Desalination of Pickled Gherkins
    (3-1968) (39) D #6

Biochemistry and Quality in Beef - Part 1
    (3-1968) (20) D #7

Manufacture of Baker's Yeasts
    (3-1968) (45) D #7

Biochemistry and Quality of Beef - Part 2
    (3-1968) (32) D #9

Ultrasonic Waves in the Concentration of Citrus Juices
    (3-1968) (25) D #10

Chocolate Manufacture
    (3-1968) (31) D #10

The Effects of Newer Forms of Packaging on the
    Microbiology and Storage Life of Meats, Poultry
    and Fish
    (7-1968) (77) C

Microbiology of Grass Silage
    (3-1968) (27) D #2

Microbiological Filtration of Liquid Sugar
    (3-1968) (58) D #9

Food Preservation - Conference Report
    (3-1968) (17) D #7

Cereal Preservation with Propionic Acid
    (3-1968) (31) D #11

Fermented Food Processes
    (4-1969) (45) D #4

Crystalline Dextrose Manufacture
    (4-1969) (19) D #7

Handling Vined Peas and Beans
    (4-1969) (26) D #7

Pneumatic Dryers for Starch and Potatoes
    (4-1969) (23) D #7

Microbiology of Margarine
    (4-1969) (31) $\underline{D}$ #7

Microwaves and Process Design
    (4-1969) (37) $\underline{D}$ #7

Contaminated Pork Products
    (4-1969) (57) $\underline{D}$ #8

Processing of Non-Newtonian Foods
    (4-1969) (15) $\underline{D}$ #10

Ice Cream Refrigeration Equipment
    (4-1969) (31) $\underline{D}$ #10

Biodeterioration of Oilseeds
    (4-1969) (57) $\underline{D}$ #10

Animal Blood Processing
    (4-1969) (15) $\underline{D}$ #12

Foods of the Future
    (4-1969) (43) $\underline{D}$ #12

Microbiology of the Hen's Eggs
    (11-1969) (245) $\underline{A}$

Industrial Aspects of Food Microbiology
    (10-1969) (39) $\underline{F}$

Industrial Microbiology and the World Food
    Problem
    (10-1969) (79) $\underline{F}$

Filtration of Edible Oils
    (4-1969) (52) $\underline{D}$ #9

Filtration in Food Processes
    (4-1969) (47) $\underline{D}$ #10

Rheology of Breadmaking
    (5-1970) (23) $\underline{D}$ #2

Egg Products
    (5-1970) (13) $\underline{D}$ #5

Tomato Powder By Spray Drying
(5-1970) (18) D #5

Glucose Syrups in Food
(5-1970) (23) D #5

Detection of Meat Odours
(5-1970) (27) D #5

Plate Heat Exchangers in Food Processing
(5-1970) (39) D #5

Chocolate - Maintaining Quality
(5-1970) (63) D #5

Mushroom in Food Technology
(5-1970) (9) D #7

Mixing Foodstuff Powders
(5-1970) (21) D #7

Emulsions in Food Technology
(5-1970) (33) D #7

Flavor and Microorganisms
(12-1970) (36) A

Food Science in India
(5-1970) (32) D #10

Protein from Green Matter
(5-1970) (37) D #10

Sauce Manufacture
(5-1970) (50) D #10

Malt Vinegar Manufacture
(5-1970) (54) D #10

Production of Tender Meat
(5-1970) (55) D #11

Clostridium Perfringens Food Poisoning
(24-1970) (359) H

Pharmaceutical Gelatin
   (5-1970) (17) D #12

Chemical Engineering in Tea Manufacture
   (5-1970) (29) D #12

Microorganisms as Potential Sources of Food
   (13-1970) (139) A

Freeze Drying Foodstuffs
   (5-1970) (23) D #6

Continuous Sterilization of Food
   (5-1970) (57) D #3

Automation of Canning Process Calculation
   (6-1971) (35) D #11

Processing Seaweed for Agar
   (6-1971) (51) D #3

Canning of Ham for Preservation
   (6-1971) (15) D #5

Manufacture of Jams, Sauces and Pickles
   (6-1971) (17) D #5

Vinegar Quality - Legal and Commercial Standards
   (6-1971) (21) D #5

Spanish Wine Vinegar
   (6-1971) (27) D #5

Biochemical Basis of Fish Freshness
   (6-1971) (36) D #5

Rheological Properties of Selected Foodstuffs
   (6-1971) (52) D #5

Packaging Biological Materials
   (6-1971) (47) D #5

Public Health Aspects of Food Processing
   (6-1971) (21) D #6

Microbial Safety in Emulsions
    (6-1971) (25) D #6

A Review of Composting - Part 1
    (6-1971) (32) D #6

Microbiology of Beet Sugar
    (6-1971) (39) D #6

Comminution in the Food Industry
    (6-1971) (51) D #6

Cryogenic Advances in Food Technology
    (6-1971) (9) D #10

Review of Composting - Part 2
    (6-1971) (26) D #10

Additives, Poisons and Convenience
    (6-1971) (3) D #12

Surfactants in Foodstuffs
    (6-1971) (11) D #12

Food Standards in the UK
    (6-1971) (13) D #12

Sweetness in Food
    (6-1971) (17) D #12

Meat Processing with Ascorbic Acid
    (6-1971) (25) D #12

Seasoning in Meat Products
    (6-1971) (27) D #12

Colouring of Food and Drinks
    (6-1971) (29) D #12

Microbial Syntheses of Proteins
    (6-1971) (41) D #2

The Microbe as A Source of Food
    (26-1972) (427) H

Modern Flour Milling
  (7-1972) (38) D #1

Mould Spoilage of Foods
  (7-1972) (11) D #5

Sausage Meat Changes in Cold Storage - 1
  (7-1972) (27) D #5

Grading Green Coffee
  (7-1972) (18) D #10

Vacuum Equipment for Evaporative Cooling
  (7-1972) (15) D #10

Caramel - Part 1 - The Browning Reactions
  (7-1972) (11) D #12

Health Foods
  (7-1972) (15) D #12

Sausage Meat Changes in Cold Storage - 2
  (7-1972) (18) D #12

Polyglycerol Esters as Food Additives
  (7-1972) (27) D #12

Views on Quality Control in Food Processing
  (8-1973) (9) D #2

Curing Meat Products
  (8-1973) (25) D #3

Modern Bread Improvers
  (8-1973) (11) D #5

Protein Enriched Bread
  (8-1973) (16) D #5

Caramel - Part 2: Manufacture, Composition and
  Properties
  (8-1973) (17) D #4

Changing Perspectives in Food Microbiology
  (14-1973) (151) F

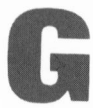

GENETICS

The Origin of Bacterial Species. Genetic Recombina-
tion and Factors Limiting it Between Bacterial
Populations
   (24-1960) (201) B

Variation in Microorganisms
   (1-1960) (207) F

The Genetics and Cytology of Chlamydomonas
   (14-1960) (197) H

Synchronous Division of Microorganisms
   (14-1960) (283) H

Gene Action
   (14-1960) (311) H

Advances in the Study of Respiration-Deficient
Mutation in Yeast and Other Microorganisms
   (25-1961) (404) B

Induced Mutagenesis in the Selection of Microorganisms
   (4-1962) (1) A

Gene Expression: Its Specificity and Regulation
     (16-1962) (1) H̲

Parasexual Phenomena in Microorganisms
     (16-1962) (35) H̲

Genetics of Bacteriophage
     (16-1962) (205) H̲

Bacterial Conjugation
     (16-1962) (289) H̲

Genetic Transformation of Rhizobium: A Review of
   the Work
     (27-1963) (228) B̲

Interspecific Hybridization in the Fungi
     (17-1963) (31) H̲

Fine Structure Genetics and Its Relationship to
   Function
     (17-1963) (49) H̲

RNA Synthesis and Turnover in Mammalian Cells Propagated
   in Vitro
     (17-1963) (139) H̲

The Genetics of Animal Viruses
     (18-1964) (47) H̲

Genetic Aspects of Metabolic Control
     (18-1964) (95) H̲

Selection, Improvement and Preservation of Microorganisms
     (5-1964) (3) C̲

Developmental Phenomena in Microorganisms and In
   Higher Forms of Life
     (19-1965) (59) H̲

Bacterial Diversity: The Natural History of Selected
   Morphologically Unusual Bacteria
     (19-1965) (407) H̲

Genetics in Applied Microbiology
(8-1966) (29) A

Regulation of Chromosome Replication and Segregation
in Bacteria
(30-1966) (3) B

Yeast Genetics
(20-1966) (151) H

Microbial Transformation and Transfection
(20-1966) (371) H

Suppression
(20-1966) (401) H

Genetic Aspects of Drug Resistance
(6-1966) (212) I

Strain Development in Industrially Important Microorganisms - Symposium
(7-1966) (61) F

Revised Linkage Map of E. coli
(31-1967) (332) B

Revised Linkage Map of Salmonella typhimurium
(31-1967) (354) B

Genetic Analysis and Genome Structure in Streptomyces
coelicolor
(31-1967) (373) B

Episomes
(21-1967) (601) H

The Effects of Ionizing Radiation on Nucleic Acids
of Bacteriophages and Bacterial Cells
(21-1967) (325) H

Molecular Basis of Mating in the Yeast Hansenula wingei
(32-1968) (139) B

Physiology and Genetics of the RNA Control Locus in
E. coli
(32-1968) (206) B

Mathematics of Microbial Populations
   (22-1968) (519) H̲

Entry and Control of Foreign Nucleic Acid
   (32-1968) (291) B̲

Antibiotic Inhibitors of the Bacterial Ribosome
   (32-1968) (493) B̲

The Life Cycle of Bacterial Ribosomes
   (2-1968) (89) E̲

The Repair of Damaged DNA in Irradiated Bacteria
   (2-1968) (173) E̲

Budding of Yeast Cells, Their Scars and Aging
   (2-1968) (143) E̲

The Plasmids of Staphylococcus aureus and Their
   Relation to Other Extrachromosomal Elements in
   Bacteria
   (2-1968) (43) E̲

Extrachromosomal Inheritance in Bacteria
   (33-1969) (210) B̲

Self Assembly of Biological Structures
   (33-1969) (302) B̲

Genetics of Pseudomonas
   (33-1969) (419) B̲

Ribosomes: Development of Some Current Ideas
   (33-1969) (445) B̲

Genetics and Chemistry of Bacterial Flagella
   (33-1969) (454) B̲

Bacterial Conjugation
   (23-1969) (69) H̲

Sequence of Bacterial Reproduction
   (23-1969) (223) H̲

UV-Induced Mutation and DNA Repair
   (23-1969) (487) H̲

E. coli Ribosomes: Recent Developments
(23-1969) (387) H

The F-Pilus of E. coli
(3-1969) (2) E

Genetic Transfer and Bacterial Taxonomy
(34-1970) (40) B

DNA of Fungi
(34-1970) (126) B

Current Linkage Map of E. coli
(34-1970) (155) B

Current Linkage Map of Salmonella typhimurium
(34-1970) (176) B

Gene Expression in Bacteria and Some Concerns About
the Misuse of Science
(34-1970) (222) B

Bacterial Ribosome
(34-1970) (228) B

Genetics of Animal Viruses
(24-1970) (297) H

Genetic Basis of Antibody Specificity
(24-1970) (335) H

DNA Restriction and Modification Mechanisms in
Bacteria
(25-1971) (153) H

Toward a Metabolic Interpretation of Genetic Recom-
bination of E. coli and Its Phages
(25-1971) (437) H

Inhibitors of Ribosome Functions
(25-1971) (487) H

Mechanism of Cell Transformation by RNA Tumor Viruses
(25-1971) (609) H

Translation of the Genome of a Ribonucleic Acid
  Bacteriophage
    (36-1972) (109) B

Genetics and Development of Industrial Strains
    (7-1972) (29) D #7

Genetic Structure and Evolution of the Incompatability
  Factors in Higher Fungi
    (36-1972) (156) B

Molecular Structure of Bacterial Plasmids
    (36-1972) (361) B

Genetics of the Proteus Group
    (26-1972) (23) H

Regulation of Chromosome Replication and the Bacterial
  Cell Cycle
    (26-1972) (347) H

RNA Virus Gene Expression and Its Control
    (26-1972) (467) H

Linkage Map of E. coli Strain K12
    (36-1972) (504) B

Pedigrees of Some Mutant Strain of E. coli K12
    (36-1972) (525) B

Linkage Map of Salmonella typhimurium
    (36-1972) (558) B

E. coli K12 F-Prime Factors, Old and New
    (36-1972) (587) B

F^+, Hfr and F' Strains of Salmonella typhimurium and
  Salmonella abony (36-1972) (608) B

GERMFREE TECHNIQUES

Germfree Animal Techniques and Their Applications
   (1-1959) (141) A

Sterile Techniques and Economic Biology
   (4-1963) (181) F

Infective Heredity of Multiple Drug Resistance in
   Bacteria
   (27-1963) (87) B

Effects of Microbes on Germfree Animals
   (7-1965) (169) A

The Gnotobiotic Animal as a Tool in the Study of
   Host Microbial Relationships
   (35-1971) (390) B

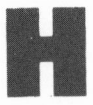

HISTORY OF MICROBIOLOGY

Louis Pasteur - Achievements and Disappointments
   (25-1961) (389) B

Biological Nitrogen Fixation - Early American Style
   (27-1963) (405) B

John Crawford and His Contributions to the Doctrine
   of Contagium Vivum
   (4-1964) (87) B

The Scientific Journal - 300th Aniversary
   (28-1964) (211) B

25 Years of Penicillin Therapy in Perspective
   (5-1965) (1) I

Thirty Years of Fermentation
   (1-1966) (9) D

The Microbiologist and His Times
   (32-1968) (401) B

Sequence in Medical History - Some Observations over
50 Years
   (23-1969) (1) H̲

Paleomicrobiology
   (23-1969) (455) H̲

Fermentation Industry - Evolution
   (4-1969) (29) D̲ #6

Some Contributions of the USDA to the Fermentation
Industry
   (13-1970) (363) A̲

Observations on Fermentation Development
   (9-1971) (113) C̲

From Protozoa to Bacteria and Viruses. Fifty Years
with Microbes
   (25-1971) (1) H̲

Dmitre Ivanovski
   (36-1972) (135) B̲

Microbiology and Fermentations in Prairie Regional
Lab. 1946 - 1971
   (15-1972) (415) A̲

HYDROCARBON FERMENTATIONS

Oxidation of Aromatic Compounds by Bacteria
   (3-1961) (193) A̲

Petroleum Microbiology
   (2-1961) (3) F̲

Microbiological Modification of Hydrocarbons
   (4-1963) (3) F̲

Microbial Degradation of Hydrocarbons
   (4-1964) (1) C̲

The Biology of Hydrocarbons
    (19-1965) (183) H̲

The Role of Microorganisms in Petroleum Exploration
    (19-1965) (351) H̲

Detergent and Hydrocarbon Oxidations
    (6-1965) (3) F̲

Hydrocarbon Deterioration
    (6-1965) (61) F̲

Methane Fermentation
    (21-1967) (121) H̲

Microbial Utilization of Methane
    (4-1969) (51) D̲ #1

Microbial Growth on C1 Compounds
    (4-1969) (25) D̲ #2

Biotransformations Using Hydrocarbons
    (4-1969) (71) D̲ #9

Microbial Protein from Petroleum
    (5-1970) (19) D̲ #6

Fermentation of Hydrocarbons
    (12-1971) (61) F̲

Utilization of Aliphatic Hydrocarbons by Microorganisms
    (5-1971) (1) E̲

Extracellular Accumulation of Metabolic Products by
  Hydrocarbon-Degrading Microorganisms
    (14-1971) (249) A̲

Methane Gas Fermentation - Technology
    (7-1972) (37) D̲ #6

Microbial Utilization of Methanol
    (15-1972) (337) A̲

The Production of Biomass from Hydrogen and Carbon
  Dioxide
    (1-1972) (143) J̲

Liquid and Solid Hydrocarbons
(1-1972) (169) J̲

IMMUNOLOGY

Antigenic Properties of Staph. aureus
   (24-1960) (374) B

Interpretation of Immunodiffusion Tests
   (14-1960) (161) H

Immunofluorescent Staining: The Fluorescent Antibody
   Method
   (25-1961) (49) B

Antigenic Variation in Unicellular Organisms
   (15-1961) (263) H

Oral Poliomyelitis Vaccine
   (25-1961) (383) B

Recent Experience with Antiviral Vaccines
   (15-1961) (297) H

Elaboration of Antibodies by Single Cells
   (16-1962) (53) H

The Nature of Antibodies and Antigens
   (16-1962) (101) H

Effects of Specific Antibodies on Tissue Cells
(16-1962) (265) H̲

Transplanted and Spontaneous Tumors
(26-1962) (336) B̲

Soviet Viable Pasteurella tularensis Vaccines
(26-1962) (354) B̲

Enzymatic and Nonenzymatic Alterations of Erythrocyte
Surface Antigens
(27-1963) (191) B̲

Symposium on Relationship of Structure of Microorganisms to Their Immunological Properties
(27-1963) (325) B̲

Basis for Immunity to Typhoid in Mice and the Question
of "Cellular Immunity"
(27-1963) (391) B̲

Methods of Immunologic Injury to Tissues
(17-1963) (263) H̲

Sensitivity to Homografts of Normal Tissues and Cells
(17-1963) (531) H̲

The Immunological Function of the Bursa of Fabricius
in the Chicken
(18-1964) (253) H̲

Fluorescent-Antibody Techniques in Diagnostic Bacteriology
(29-1965) (222) B̲

Complement
(19-1965) (285) H̲

The Immune Globulins
(19-1965) (301) H̲

Phagocytosis
(19-1965) (339) H̲

Infectious Disease and Immune Mechanisms
(5-1965) (22) I̲

Macrophage Function in Infectious Disease with Inbred
  Rabbits
    (29-1965) (466) B

Immunochemistry of O & R Antigens of Salmonella and
  Related Enterobacteriaceae
    (30-1966) (192) B

Symposium on in Vitro Studies of the Immune Response
    (30-1966) (383) B

Blood Groups, Disease and Selection
    (30-1966) (427) B

Interferon
    (20-1966) (291) H

Tumor Antigens
    (20-1966) (223) H

Mechanisms by Which Antibiotics Increase the Incidence and Severity of Candiasis and Alter the
  Immunological Defenses
    (30-1966) (442) B

Experimentally Induced Immunity in the Mycoses
    (31-1967) (35) B

Interferon Induction with Statolon in the Intact
  Animal
    (31-1967) (132) B

Various Molecular Species of Interferon Induced by
  Viral and Nonviral Agents
    (31-1967) (138) B

Cellular Resistance to Induction of Interferon
    (31-1967) (145) B

Antibody Heterogeneity and Serological Reactions
    (31-1967) (157) B

Cellular Commitments to Immune Responses
    (21-1967) (181) H

Salmonella 0 Antigens and Virulence
(21-1967) (443) H

Tolerance
(21-1967) (157) H

Antiserum Production in Experimental Animals
(9-1967) (39) A

Production of Virus Vaccines
(2-1967) (25) D #12

Cellular Hypersensitivity and Cellular Immunity in
the Pathogenesis of Tuberculosis
(32-1968) (85) B

Histamine-Sensitizing Factors from Microbial Agents
(32-1968) (103) B

Biochemical Challenge of Microbial Pathogenicity
(32-1968) (164) B

On the Mechanism of Immunity - In Defense of Evolution
(22-1968) (283) H

Affinity of Antigen for White Cells and Its Relation
to the Induction of Antibody Formation
(32-1968) (404) B

Immunoglobulins and Immunocytes
(33-1969) (159) B

Induction of Antibodies
(23-1969) (199) H

Immuno-Electrophoresis
(4-1969) (38) D #8

Foot and Mouth Disease Vaccine
(4-1969) (49) D #6

Fractionation of Human Plasma
(5-1970) (23) D #10

Immunological Methods in Industry
(5-1970) (47) D #11

Immunological Enrichment as Studied by Cell Culture
Techniques
(24-1970) (373) H

Genetic Basis of Antibody Specificity
(24-1970) (335) H

Endogenous Broncho-Active Substances and Their
Antagonism
(5-1970) (95) G

The Role of Slow Reacting Substance in Asthma
(5-1970) (109) G

Newer Techniques in Virus Vaccine Production
(11-1970) (3) F

Serotype Expression in Paramecium
(4-1970) (132) E

Chemical Markers of Transplantation Individually
Solubilized with Sonic Energy
(35-1971) (59) B

Immunochemistry of Shigella flexneri O-Antigens: A
Study of Structural and Genetic Aspects of the Biosyntheses of Cell Surface Antigens
(35-1971) (117) B

Immunological Paralysis of Mice with Pneumococcal
Polysaccharide Antigens
(35-1971) (267) B

Macrophage-Cytophilic Antibodies and the Function
of Macrophage-Bound Immunoglobulins
(35-1971) (365) B

Destruction of Virus Infected Cells by Immunological
Mechanisms
(25-1971) (283) H

Isolation of Lymphoid Cells with Active Surface Re-
ceptor Sites
(25-1971) (291) H

INSECTICIDES (MICROBIAL)

Symposium on Microbial Insecticides
   (29-1965) (364) <u>B</u>

Crystal-Forming Bacteria as Insect Pathogens
   (8-1966) (291) <u>A</u>

Insecticides of Crystal Forming Bacteria
   (4-1969) (29) <u>D</u> #12

Bacillus thurengiensis: Microbiological Considera-
tions
   (23-1969) (357) <u>H</u>

Insecticidal Activity of Microbial Metabolite
   (9-1971) (79) <u>C</u>

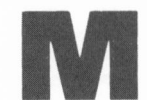

MEDICAL MICROBIOLOGY

The 1959 Fort Detrick Symposium on Nonspecific Resistance to Infections (18 Papers-192 pp.)
    (24-1960) (1-192) B

Factors Influencing the Occurrence of Illness During
Naturally Acquired Poliomyelitis Cirus Infections
    (24-1960) (341) B

The Arthropod-Borne Viruses of Man and Other Animals
    (14-1960) (261) H

Intramural Spread of Bacteria and Viruses in Human
Populations
    (14-1960) (43) H

Infectious Diseases - I
    (1-1961) (1) I

Infectious Diseases - II
    (1-1961) (100) I

The Histotoxic Clostridial Infects of Man
    (26-1962) (177) B

Infectious Diseases - I
  (2-1962) (1) I

Infectious Diseases - II
  (2-1962) (76) I

Clinical Evaluation - I
  (2-1962) (318) I

Clinical Evaluation - II
  (2-1962) (384) I

Clinical Evaluation - III
  (2-1962) (476) I

Healthy Carriage of Staphylococcus aureus: Its
  Prevalence and Importance
  (27-1963) (56) B

The Inflammatory Response
  (27-1963) (117) B

Coccidiosis
  (17-1963) (179) H

Toxoplasma and Toxoplasmosis
  (17-1963) (429) H

Pathogenic "Atypical" Mycobacteria
  (17-1963) (473) H

Infectious Diseases
  (3-1963) (604) I

Clinical - General
  (3-1963) (714) I

Metabolism of Microorganisms as Related to Their
  Pathogenecity
  (17-1963) (297) H

Present Status of the El Tor vibrio Problem
  (28-1964) (72) B

Agents of Trachoma and Inclusion Conjunctivitis
  (18-1964) (301) H

Infectious Diseases
   (4-1964) (632) I

Experimental Infections
   (4-1964) (733) I

Borreliae, Human Relapsing Fever, and Parasite-
Vector-Host Relationships
   (29-1965) (46) B

Escherichia coli and Neonatal Disease of Calves
   (29-1965) (75) B

Oral Microbiology
   (8-1966) (195) A

Roles of Metallic Ions in Host-Parasite Interactions
   (30-1966) (136) B

Listeria monocytogenes and Listeric Infections
   (30-1966) (309) B

Infectious Diseases - Experimental Studies in Animals
and Humans
   (6-1966) (6) I

Clinical Evaluation of Antimicrobial Agents in Humans
   (6-1966) (42) I

Comparative Ecology of Respiratory Mycotic Disease
Agents
   (31-1967) (6) B

Epidemiological Aspects of Respiratory Mycotic
Infections
   (31-1967) (25) B

The Possible Role of Microorganisms and Viruses in
the Etiology of Chronic Degenerative Diseases of
Man
   (21-1967) (467) H

Food Borne Salmonellosis
   (21-1967) (495) H

Defenses Against Biological Warfare
   (21-1967) (639) H

Practical Aspects of Mycoplasmoses of Man and Animals
   (8-1967) (35) F

Round Table - The Regulation of Clinical Investiga-
tion
   (7-1967) (10) I

Infectious Diseases: Experimental and Clinical
Studies
   (7-1967) (40) I

Round Table: Optimal Duration of Antibiotic Therapy
in Severe Bacterial Infections
   (7-1967) (183) I

Phylogenetic Relationships of Drug-Resistance Factors and Other Transmissible Bacterial Plasmids
   (32-1968) (55) B

The Ecology of Transferable Drug Resistance in the
Enterobacteria
   (22-1968) (131) H

Foot and Mouth Disease
   (22-1968) (201) H

Dental Caries and Peridontal Disease Considered as
Infectious Diseases
   (11-1969) (135) A

Chemotherapy of the Drug Resistant Malarias
   (23-1969) (427) H

Chemotherapy and the Control of Infections in Man
   (9-1969) (352) I

Control of Infectious Diseases
   (9-1969) (1) I

Therapeutic Dentrifices
   (13-1970) (343) A

Infectious Disease and Social Change
   (10-1970) I̲

The Control of Infections in Humans
   (10-1970) I̲

Experimental Studies of Infection in Animals and
   Humans
   (10-1970) I̲

Vibrio cholerae Enterotoxin and Its Mode of Action
   (35-1971) (1) B̲

Diseases of Oysters
   (25-1971) (211) H̲

Stomach Microbiology of Primates
   (25-1971) (429) H̲

Emerging Diseases of Man and Animals
   (25-1971) (465) H̲

Pathogenecity of the L-Phase of Bacteria
   (26-1972) (55) H̲

Current Problems and Approaches in Skin Microbiology
   (14-1973) (125) F̲

MICROBIOCIDES

Factors Affecting the Antimicrobial Activity of
   Phenols
   (1-1959) (123) A̲

Fungal Metabolism and Fungicides
   (1-1960) (169) F̲

Correlations Between Microbiological Morphology and
   the Chemistry of Biocides
   (5-1963) (1) A̲

Biocides in Industry
   (2-1967) (13) D #11

Bacteriocides in Dairies
   (2-1967) (21) D #11

Quaternary Ammonium Compounds
   (2-1967) (33) D #11

Phenolic-Anionic Detergent Systems
   (2-1967) (26) D #11

Antibacterials in Soaps
   (8-1967) (1) F

Chemical Sterilization
   (8-1968) (141) C

Chemical Sterilizers
   (10-1968) (291) A

Assessment of Industrial Biocides
   (3-1968) (23) D #11

Biocides in Bulk Milk Tank Cleaning
   (3-1968) (27) D #11

Fungal Growth in a Bonded Warehouse
   (3-1968) (35) D #11

Control of Site Contamination
   (3-1968) (37) D #11

Disinfection in Fermentation Laboratories
   (4-1969) (15) D #11

Plant Hygiene in Biochemical Processes
   (4-1969) (19) D #11

Biocides for Food Plant
   (4-1969) (23) D #11

Dosing Equipment for Biocides
   (4-1969) (31) D #11

MUSHROOM CULTURE

O

ORGANIC ACIDS

P

The Biosynthesis and Interconversion of Purines and
   Their Derivatives
      (24-1960) (309) <u>B</u>

Fungal Metabolism and Fungicides
      (1-1960) (169) <u>F</u>

Microbial Nutrition
      (14-1960) (17) <u>H</u>

Protein Synthesis in Microorganisms
      (14-1960) (65) <u>H</u>

Energy Metabolism in Chemolithotropic Bacteria
      (14-1960) (83) <u>H</u>

Enzyme Localization in Bacteria
      (14-1960) (241) <u>H</u>

Nutrition, Metabolism and Pathogenicity of Mycoplasmas
      (14-1960) <u>H</u>

Photosynthetic Mechanisms in Bacteria and Plants
      (25-1961) (1) <u>B</u>

An Introduction to the Origin and Biochemistry of
   Microbial Halometabolites
      (25-1961) (111) <u>B</u>

Physiology of the Actinomycetes
      (15-1961) (1) <u>H</u>

Interactions Between Pesticides and Soil Microorganisms
      (15-1961) (69) <u>H</u>

Sugar Transport in Microorganisms
      (15-1961) (197) <u>H</u>

Metabolism of C_1 Compounds in Autotrophic and
   Heterotrophic Microorganisms
      (15-1961) (119) <u>H</u>

Symposium on Metabolism of Inorganic Compounds
      (26-1962) (14) <u>B</u>

Chemical Composition and Metabolism of Protozoa
(17-1963) (451) H

The Present Status of the 2,3,Butylene Glycol Fermentation
(5-1963) (135) A

Secondary Factors in Fermentation Processes
(6-1964) (69) A

Microbial Formation and Degradation of Minerals
(6-1964) (153) A

Comparative Physiology of Pleuropneumonia-Like
and L-Type Organisms
(28-1964) (97) B

Some Aspects of the Endogenous Metabolism of Bacteria
(28-1964) (126) B

Oxidation of Aliphatic Glycols by Acetic Acid
Bacteria
(28-1964) (164) B

Aspects of Bacterial Response to the Ionic Environment
(28-1964) (296) B

Responses of Microorganisms to Sterols and Steroids
(18-1964) (167) H

Biochemical Ecology of Soil Microorganisms
(18-1964) (217) H

Effects of Hydrostatic Pressure on Microbial
Systems
(28-1964) (14) B

Microbial Processes for Preparation of Radioactive
Compounds
(6-1964) (27) A

Preparation of Alkaloids by Saprophytic Culture of
Ergot Fungi
(5-1964) (203) C

Genetics of Metabolic Control
(18-1964) (95) H

Biodegradation: Problems of Molecular Recalcitrance
and Microbial Fallibility
(7-1965) (35) A

Microbial Production of Metal-Organic Compounds
and Complexes
(7-1965) (103) A

Nutrition of Systemic and Subcutaneous Pathogenic
Fungi
(29-1965) (397) B

Movement and Locomotion of Microorganisms
(19-1965) (21) H

Industrial Fermentations and Their Relation to
Regulatory Mechanisms
(8-1966) (1) A

The Tricarboxylic Acid Cycle
(1-1966) (465) D

Roles of Amino Acid Activating Enzymes in Cellular
Physiology
(30-1966) (701) B

Inorganic Polyphosphates in Biology: Structure,
Metabolism and Function
(30-1966) (772) B

Biosynthesis of Lipids in Microorganisms
(20-1966) (13) H

The Biosynthesis of Bacterial Polysaccharides
(20-1966) (253) H

Microbiology of Paper and Pulp Symposium
(7-1966) (173) F

Regulation of Nucleic Acid and Protein Formation in
Bacteria
(1-1967) (39) F

Biochemical Aspects of Extreme Halophilism
(1-1967) (97) F

The Biochemistry of the Bacterial Endospore
(1-1967) (133) F

Bacterial Phosphatides and Natural Relationships
(31-1967) (54) B

Biodynamic Effects of Oligonucleotides
(31-1967) (83) B

Extracellular Lipids of Yeasts
(31-1967) (194) B

Arrangement of Base Sequences in DNA
(31-1967) (215) B

DNA of the Blue-Green Algae
(31-1967) (315) B

Fatty Acid Synthesis and Metabolism in Microorganisms
(21-1967) (225) H

Mechanisms of Nucleic Acid Synthesis
(21-1967) (369) H

Mechanisms of Protein Synthesis
(21-1967) (383) H

Microbial Models of Tumor Metabolism
(9-1967) (69) A

Cellulose and Celluloysis
(9-1967) (91) A

Microbiological Aspects of the Formation and
Degradation of Cellulosic Fibers
(9-1967) (131) A

The Biotransformation of Lignin to Humus - Facts
and Postulates
(9-1967) (171) A

Temperature Effects Upon Microorganisms
(21-1967) (101) H

Survival of Bacteria
   (21-1967) (143) H̲

Alternate Pathways of Metabolism of Short Chain
   Fatty Acids
   (32-1968) (1) B̲

Protein Synthesizing Machinery of Thermophilic
   Bacteria
   (32-1968) (27) B̲

Fatty Acid Oxidation
   (3-1968) (33) D̲ #6

Anaplerotic Pathways of Metabolism
   (3-1968) (40) D̲ #8

Photochemical and Electron Transport Reactions of
   Bacterial Photosynthesis
   (32-1968) (243) B̲

RNA from Animal Cells
   (32-1968) (262) B̲

Cell Wall Chemistry, Morphogenesis and Taxonomy of
   Fungi
   (22-1968) (87) H̲

Biochemical Peculiarities of Trypanosomatid Flagel-
   lates
   (22-1968) (109) H̲

Bacterial Cytochromes
   (22-1968) (181) H̲

Energy-Coupling Mechanisms in Chemolithoropic
   Bacteria
   (22-1968) (489) H̲

Pathways of Biosynthesis of Aromatic Amino Acids
   and Vitamins and Their Control in Microorganisms
   (32-1968) (465) B̲

Microbiological Transformations of Sugars and Related
   Compounds
   (7-1968) (177) C̲

Microbial Corrosion
   (3-1968) (17) D #12

The Bacterial Photosynthetic Apparatus
   (2-1968) (1) E

Dextran-Manufacture and Use - Part 1
   (3-1968) (15) D #2

Dextran-Manufacture and Use - Part 2
   (3-1968) (55) D #3

Production of Purine Nucleotides by Fermentation
   (8-1968) (35) C

Synthetic Sugar Polymers
   (3-1968) (31) D #12

Molecular Aspects of Endotoxic Reactions
   (33-1969) (72) B

Microbial Fermentation of Lower Terpenoids
   (4-1969) (50) D #2

Mechanism of Protein Biosynthesis
   (33-1969) (264) B

Regulation of Enzyme Function
   (23-1969) (47) H

Kinetics of Nutrient Limited Growth
   (23-1969) (473) H

Total Synthesis of Acetate from CO_2 by Heterotrophic
   Bacteria
   (23-1969) (515) H

Carbohydrate Metabolism in Microorganisms
   (23-1969) (539) H

The Roles of Exogenous Organic Matter in the Physiology
   of Chemolithrotropic Bacteria
   (3-1969) (159) E

Microbial Production of Phenazines
(13-1970) (267) <u>A</u>

Metabolism of Acylanilide Herbicides
(13-1970) (317) <u>A</u>

Progress Report on Microbial Polysaccharides
(11-1970) (81) <u>F</u>

Microbial Metabolites as Potentially Useful Pharma-
cologically Active Agents
(12-1970) (277) <u>A</u>

Biosynthesis of Secondary Metabolites - Roles of
Trace Minerals
(4-1970) (1) <u>E</u>

Catabolite Repression and Other Control Mechanisms
in Carbohydrate Utilization
(4-1970) (252) <u>E</u>

Roles of Lipids in the Biosynthesis of the Bacterial
Cell Envelope
(35-1971) (14) <u>B</u>

Microbial Growth Rates in Nature
(35-1971) (39) <u>B</u>

Regulation of Catabolic Pathways in Pseudomonas
(35-1971) (87) <u>B</u>

Biochemical and Physiological Aspects of Differentiation in the Fungi
(5-1971) (45) <u>E</u>

High Energy Elections in Bacteria
(5-1971) (135) <u>E</u>

Branched Election-Transport Systems in Bacteria
(5-1971) (173) <u>E</u>

Generation and Utilization of Energy During Growth
(5-1971) (213) <u>E</u>

Catabolism of Aromatic Compounds by Microorganisms
(6-1971) (1) <u>E</u>

Conservation and Transformation of Energy by Bacterial Membranes
        (36-1972) (172) B

Dinitrogen (N_2) Fixation (With a Biochemical Emphasis)
        (36-1972) (231) B

Minerals Microbiology
        (13-1972) (57) F

Turnover of Intracellular Protein
        (26-1972) (103) H

Production of Volatile Sulfur Compounds by Microorganisms
        (26-1972) (127) H

Ferredoxins and Flavodoxins of Bacteria
        (26-1972) (139) H

Biogenesis of Mitochondria in Microorganisms
        (26-1972) (163) H

Lipids of Protozoa: Phospholipids and Neutral
   Lipids
        (26-1972) (249) H

Inorganic Nutrition
        (26-1972) (313) H

Peptidoglycan Types of Bacterial Cell Walls and
   Their Taxonomic Implications
        (36-1972) (407) B

Bacterial Surface Translocation - A Survey and a
   Classification
        (36-1972) (478) B

Effects of Environment on Bacterial Wall Content
   and Composition
        (7-1972) (83) E

Metabolism of 1-Carbon Compounds by Microorganisms
        (7-1972) (119) E

PLANT DISEASE

Status of Antibiotics in Plant Disease Control
(1-1959) (87) <u>A</u>

Plant Nematode Interrelationships
(15-1961) (177) <u>H</u>

Dwart Bunt of Wheat
(17-1963) (199) <u>H</u>

Microbial Toxins in Plant Disease
(17-1963) (223) <u>H</u>

Antibiotics in Control of Plant Disease
(17-1963) (243) <u>H</u>

Phytotoxic Substances from Soil Microorganisms and
  Crop Residues
  (28-1964) (181) <u>B</u>

Resistance of Plants to Infectious Agents
  (20-1966) (337) <u>H</u>

Unusual Vectors of Plant Viruses
(21-1967) (205) <u>H</u>

Antibiotics in Control of Plant Pathogens
(10-1968) (313) <u>A</u>

The Genus Erwinia: Enterobacteria Pathogenic to
  Plants and Animals
  (26-1972) (389) <u>H</u>

POLYSACCHARIDES (MICROBIAL)

Dextran - Manufacture and Use - Part 1
(3-1968) (15) <u>D</u> #2

Dextran - Manufacture and Use - Part 2
   (3-1968) (55) D #3

Microbial Exopolysaccharides - Potential
   (7-1972) (27) D #11

Fermentation of Polysaccharide Gums
   (8-1973) (33) D #1

PRESERVATION TECHNIQUES

Preservation of Foods and Drugs by Ionizing Radiations
   (1-1959) (49) A

Preservation of Bacteria by Lyophilization
   (3-1961) (1) A

Preservation of Oil-in-Water Systems
   (3-1962) (265) F

The Preservation of Cultures
   (4-1964) (189) C

The Microbiology of Freeze Dried Foods
   (7-1965) (305) A

Low Temperature Microbiology
   (7-1965) (335) A

Nisin and Food Preservation
   (1-1966) (461) D

Viability Measurements and the Survival of Microbes
   Under Minimum Stress
   (1-1967) (1) F

Cryogenic Storage Vessels
   (2-1967) (29) D #7

Air Blast Freezing of Fish
   (2-1967) (42) D #6

The Inclusion of Antimicrobial Agents in Pharmaceutical Products
   (9-1967) (1) A

Bacteriology of Fish Spoilage and Preservation
   (6-1967) (169) C

Freeze Drying Biological Materials - Part 1
   (3-1968) (11) D #6

Food Preservation - Conference Report
   (3-1968) (17) D #7

Freeze Drying Biological Materials - Part 2
   (3-1968) (48) D #7

Heat and Mass Transfer in Freeze Drying
   (3-1968) (59) D #11

Storage of Biological Materials
   (4-1969) (11) D #10

Freeze-Drying Foodstuffs
   (5-1970) (23) D #6

Storage of Biological Materials
   (5-1970) (13) D #10

Product Survey - Cryogenics and Refrigeration
   (5-1970) (29) D #10

Canning of Ham for Preservation
   (6-1971) (15) D #5

Meat Processing with Ascorbic Acid
   (6-1971) (25) D #12

Preservation of Microorganisms
   (7-1972) (24) D #7

PROSTAGLANDINS

Commentary - Prostaglandins - Synthesis or Fermentation
    (7-1972) (3) D #3

PROTOZOA

Microbial Ecology of the Rumen
  (24-1960) (353) B

Fine Structure of Protozoa
  (15-1961) (47) H

Plant Nematode Interrelationships
  (15-1961) (177) H

Chemical Composition and Metabolism of Protozoa
  (17-1963) (451) H

The Rumen Bacteria and Protozoa
  (18-1964) (131) H

Industrial Aspects of Protozoology
  (6-1965) (61) F

Structure and Function of Protozoa
  (20-1966) (131) H

Antiparasitic Agents
  (8-1967) (117) F

Rumen Microbes
  (4-1969) (53) D #11

Encystment in Amoebae
  (4-1970) (106) E

Serotype Expression in Paramecium
    (4-1970) (132) $\underline{E}$

Biology of Large Amoeba
    (25-1971) (27) $\underline{H}$

Pathogenicity of Soil Amoeba
    (25-1971) (231) $\underline{H}$

S

SINGLE CELL PROTEIN

Potential for Increasing Food Production through
  Microbiology
    (29-1965) (251) <u>B</u>

Microorganisms as Potential Food Sources
    (7-1966) (203) <u>F</u>

Industrial Microbiology and the World Food Problem
    (10-1969) (79) <u>F</u>

Foods of the Future
    (4-1969) (43) <u>D</u> #12

Microorganisms as Potential Sources of Food
    (13-1970) (139) <u>A</u>

Microbial Protein from Petroleum
    (5-1970) (19) <u>D</u> #6

Microbial Synthesis of Proteins
    (6-1971) (41) <u>D</u> #2

SCP from Hydrocarbons
    (7-1972) (31) <u>D</u> #5

The Microbe as a Source of Food
   (26-1972) (427) H̲

Recent Advances in Protein Production
   (8-1973) (31) D̲ #2

Prediction of Substrate Yield Coefficients
   (8-1973) (13) D̲ #4

Methanol-Bacterium Process for SCP
   (8-1973) (22) D̲ #6

SOIL MICROBIOLOGY

Biochemical Pathways in Legume Root Nodule Nitrogen
   Fixation
   (24-1960) (246) B̲

Interactions Between Pesticides and Soil Microorganisms
   (15-1961) (69) H̲

The Bacteroids of the Genus Rhizobium
   (26-1962) (119) B̲

Nitrogen Fixation - Role of Ferredoxin in Anaerobic
   Metabolism
   (17-1963) (115) H̲

Biochemical Ecology of Soil Microorganisms
   (18-1964) (217) H̲

Interactions Between Plant Roots and Soil Microorganisms
   (19-1965) (241) H̲

Biotransformation of Lignin to Humus - Fact and
   Postulates
   (9-1967) (171) A̲

Peat Microbiology
(4-1969) (47) D #11

Rhizobia
(23-1969) (137) H

The Physiology of Ectotrophic Mycorrhizos
(3-1969) (53) E

The Pathways of Nitrogen Fixation
(8-1972) (59) E

SOLVENTS

The Acetone-Butanol Fermentation
(3-1961) (71) C

SPACE MICROBIOLOGY

Space Age Microbiology
(1-1960) (13) F

Microbiological Applications for Space Vehicles
and Extraterrestrial Stations
(3-1962) (1) F

Space Microbiology
(4-1964) (183) F

Space Microbiology
(9-1968) (19) F

Detection of Life in Soil on Earth and Other Planets
(10-1968) (1) A

For What Shall We Search
(10-1968) (5) <u>A</u>

Relevance of Soil Microbiology to Search for Life
on Other Planets
(10-1968) (17) <u>A</u>

Experiments and Instrumentation for Extraterrestrial Life Detection
(10-1968) (55) <u>A</u>

STATISTICS AND EXPERIMENTAL DESIGN

Non Linear Problems in Statistical and Mathematical
Interpretation
(2-1960) (71) <u>C</u>

STERILIZATION

Sterilization of Media for Biochemical Processes
(2-1960) (313) <u>A</u>

Self-Sanitizing Agents for Fabrics
(1-1960) (57) <u>F</u>

Air Sterilization
(2-1960) (302) <u>A</u>

Gaseous Sterilization
(15-1961) (245) <u>H</u>

The Sterilization of Air
(4-1964) (35) <u>C</u>

Modern Trends in Steam Sterilization
(5-1964) (237) <u>C</u>

Microbiological Aspects of Radiation Sterilization
(5-1964) (238) C

Kinetics of the Inactivation of Viruses
(28-1964) (150) B

Cold Sterilization Techniques
(7-1965) (81) A

Independent-Action and Birth-Death Models in Experimental Microbiology
(29-1965) (102) B

Fermentor Mash Sterilization
(1-1966) (41) D

Ultra-High Temperature Treatment of Milk
(1-1966) (103) D

Package Boilers
(1-1966) (109) D

Evaluating Pasteurization Processes
(1-1966) (121) D

Filtration-Sterilization of Air and Gases
(1-1966) (177) D

Sterilization Processes and Problems
(1-1966) (268) D

Radiation Sterilization of Meat
(1-1966) (487) D

Filtration-Sterilization of Beverages
(1-1966) (470) D

Thermal Death Rate of Bacterial Spore
(2-1967) (35) D #2

Air Sterilization with Fibrous Filters
(2-1967) (21) D #9

Chemical Sterilization
(8-1968) (141) C

Chemical Sterilizers
   (10-1968) (291) $\underline{A}$

UV Lamps for Disinfection
   (4-1969) (27) $\underline{D}$ #11

Continuous Sterilization of Food
   (5-1970) (57) $\underline{D}$ #3

Mechanisms of Thermal Drying in Nonsporulating
  Bacteria
   (12-1970) (89) $\underline{A}$

Air Sterilization and Disinfection
   (5-1970) (21) $\underline{D}$ #9

Sterilization of Industrial Water
   (5-1970) (25) $\underline{D}$ #9

Pasteurization and Sterilization of Sludges
   (5-1970) (44) $\underline{D}$ #9

Bacterial Filtration of Air
   (5-1970) (47) $\underline{D}$ #5

Cleaning and Sterilizing in Brewing
   (5-1970) (41) $\underline{D}$ #4

Continuous Sterilization of Food
   (5-1970) (57) $\underline{D}$ #3

Sterile and Ultra Pure Water for Pharmaceutical
  Processes
   (7-1972) (17) $\underline{D}$ #7

Recent Approaches to Sterilization and Achievement
  of Sterility
   (14-1973) (3) $\underline{F}$

STEROIDS

The Microbiological Transformation of Steroids
(2-1960) (183) A

The Metabolism of Cardiac Lactones by Microorganisms
(3-1961) (279) A

Microbiological Processing of Steroids
(1-1966) (201) D

Transformation of Organic Compounds by Fungal Spores
(10-1968) (221) A

SUGAR PRODUCTION

Starch Conversion Processes
(1-1966) (49) D

Microbiology in Sugar Production
(1-1966) (284) D

Wet Maize Milling
(1-1966) (318) D

Crystalline Dextrose Manufacture
(4-1969) (19) D #7

Starch Refining 1 - Processing
(5-1970) (38) D #6

Starch Refining 2 - Quality, Yields and Equipment
(5-1970) (30) D #7

Phosphate Content in Glucose Syrup Conversion
(7-1972) (25) D #7

T

TAXONOMIC GROUPS OF MICROORGANISMS

The Morphology and Natural Relationships of Saprophytic Actinomycetes
(1-1959) (29) C

The Lactobacilli - I
(2-1960) (1) C

The Economic Activities of Sulfate-Reducing Bacteria
(2-1960) (47) C

Microbial Ecology of the Rumen
(24-1960) (353) B

A Review of the Genus Candida
(24-1960) (397) B

Hallucinogenic Fungi
(1-1960) (109) F

Variation in Phytopathogenic Fungi
(14-1960) (1) H

Numerical Taxonomy
(4-1964) (151) F

Conservation of Microorganisms
(18-1964) (1) H

Pseudomonas and Related Genera
(18-1964) (17) H

Morphogenesis of Bacterial Aggregations
(18-1964) (111) H

The Rumen Bacteria and Protozoa
(18-1964) (131) H

New Approaches to Bacterial Taxonomy: Use of
  Computors
(18-1964) (335) H

Development of Coding Schemes for Microbial Taxonomy
(7-1965) (139) A

The Question of the Existence of Specific Marine
  Bacteria
(29-1965) (9) B

Mycoplasma Species of Man
(29-1965) (185) B

Classification of the Spore-Forming Sulfate-
  Reducing Bacteria
(29-1965) (359) B

Recent Advances in the Study of the Sulfate-
  Reducing Bacteria
(29-1965) (425) B

Flagellation as a Criteria for the Classification
  of Bacteria
(29-1965) (442) B

Lichens
(19-1965) (1) H

Pleuropneumonia-Like Organisms and Related Forms
(19-1965) (379) H

Host-Dependent Microbes
(30-1966) (114) B

Bacterial Taxonomy: A Critique
(30-1966) (257) B

Classification of Desulfovibrio Species, the
Nonsporulating Sulfate-Reducing Bacteria
(30-1966) (732) B

Biology of the Myxobacteria
(20-1966) (75) H

The Relation of the Psittacosis Group to Bacteria
and Viruses
(20-1966) (107) H

Micro-organisms of Cured Tobacco
(2-1967) (12) D #1

Problems in Taxonomy of Streptomycetes
(2-1967) (20) D #1

Euglenida/Euglenophyta
(21-1967) (31) H

Biology of Actinomycetes
(21-1967) (71) H

Photosynthetic Bacteria
(21-1967) (285) H

Identification of Yeasts
(3-1968) (32) D #5

Halophilic Bacteria
(10-1968) (73) A

Proteins and Enzymes as Taxonomic Tools
(10-1968) (137) A

Rumen Microorganisms
(4-1969) (53) D #11

Cytodifferentiation and Morphogenesis in Schizo-
phyllum commune
  (33-1969) (505) B

Micromonospora Taxonomy
  (11-1969) (101) A

Structure, Physiology and Biochemistry of Chryso-
phyceae
  (23-1969) (29) H

Rhizobia (with Particular Reference to Relationship
with Host Plants)
  (23-1969) (137) H

New Approaches to Bacterial Taxonomy: Perspective
and Prospects
  (23-1969) (239) H

Rickettsiae (as Organisms)
  (23-1969) (275) H

Structure and Function in Mycoplasma
  (23-1969) (317) H

Sugar-Fermenting Sarcinae
  (34-1970) (82) B

Saprophytic Coryneform Bacteria
  (5-1970) (209) H

Corynebacterium diphtheriae and Its Relatives
  (34-1970) (378) B

Chemotaxonomic Relationships Among Basidiomycetes
  (13-1970) (1) A

Proton Magnetic Resonance Spectroscopy - an Aid
in Identification and Chemotaxonomy of Yeasts
  (13-1970) (25) A

Genetic Transfer and Bacterial Taxonomy
  (34-1970) (40) B

Purification and Properties of Unicellular Blue-
Green Algae
   (35-1971) (171) B

Mycoplasmas and Cell Cultures
   (35-1971) (206) B

Rumen Microorganisms
   (9-1971) (41) C

Chemical Composition as a Criterion in the Classification of Actinomycetes
   (14-1971) (47) A

Biochemical Activities of Nocardia
   (14-1971) (93) A

Aggregation and Differentiation in the Cellular
Slime Molds
   (25-1971) (75) H

Prosthecate Bacteria
   (25-1971) (93) H

The Bdellovibrios
   (25-1971) (649) H

Cell Biology of the Mycoplasmas
   (36-1972) (263) B

The Genus Erwinia: Enterobacteria Pathogenic to
Plants and Animals
   (26-1972) (389) H

Physiology of the Bdellovibrios
   (8-1972) (215) E

Biology of the Bifidobacteria
   (37-1973) (136) B

TISSUE CULTURE

Large Scale Use of Animal Cell Cultures
   (3-1961) (109) A

Maintenance and Loss in Tissue Culture of Specific
Cell Characteristics
   (4-1962) (117) A

Submerged Growth of Plant Cells
   (4-1962) (213) A

Cultural Characterization of Animal Cells
   (16-1962) (141) H

Sterile Techniques and Economic Biology
   (4-1963) (181) F

RNA Synthesis and Turnover in Mammalian Cells
Propagated in Vitro
   (17-1963) (139) H

Growth of Animal Cells in Tissue Culture
   (4-1964) (61) C

Multiplication of Measles Virus in Cell Cultures
   (30-1966) (152) B

The Mammalian Cell as Differentiated Microorganisms
   (21-1967) (573) H

Tissue Culture as a Fermentation Process
   (2-1967) (42) D #4

Tissue Culture as Biochemical Tools
   (3-1968) (15) D #1

Multi Layer Perfusion Tissue Culture
   (5-1970) (21) D #3

Large Scale Cultivation of Mammalian Cells
   (13-1970) (91) A

Immunological Enrichment as Studied by Cell Culture
Techniques
(24-1970) (373) H

Mass Cultivation of Mammalian Cells
(6-1971) (15) D #7

Industrial Potential of Plant Cell Culture
(9-1971) (13) C

Insect Tissue Culture
(15-1972) (157) A

Metabolites from Animal and Plant Cell Culture
(15-1972) (215) A

TOXINS

Symposium on Bacterial Endotoxins
(25-1961) (427) B

Bacteriocins and Bacteriocin-Like Substances
(26-1962) (108) B

Phytotoxic Substances from Soil Microorganisms
and Crop Residues
(28-1964) (181) B

Mycotoxins in Feeds and Foods
(8-1966) (315) A

The Murine Toxin of Pasteurella pestis: A Study
in Its Development
(30-1966) (177) B

Chemical Nature and Biological Effects of the
Aflatoxins
(30-1966) (460) B

Biological Effects of Aflatoxin in Cell Culture
(30-1966) (471) B

Toxins Other Than Aflatoxins Produced by Aspergillus
  flavus
    (30-1966) (478) B

Aflatoxin Formation by Aspergillus flavus
    (30-1966) (795) B

Aflatoxins
    (1-1967) (25) F

Status of Bacterial Toxins and Their Nomenclature:
  Need for Discipline and Clarity of Expression
    (31-1967) (95) B

Formation and Mode of Action of Algal Toxins
    (31-1967) (180) B

Cholera Toxins
    (22-1968) (245) H

Toxins Produced by Fungi
    (22-1968) (269) H

Mycotoxins
    (7-1968) (149) C

Mycotoxins
    (10-1968) (155) A

Sporulation and the Production of Antibiotics,
  Exoenzymes and Exotoxins
    (33-1969) (48) B

Vibrio Cholera Enterotoxin and Its Mode of Action
    (35-1971) (1) B

Botulinal Toxins and the Problem of Nomenclature
  of Simple Toxins
    (35-1971) (242) B

Carcinogens Produced by Fungi
    (26-1972) (279) H

V

VINEGAR

VIRUSES

In Vitro Cell-Virus Relationships Resulting in
Cell Death
(14-1960) (177) <u>H</u>

Fine Structure of Virus-Infected Cells
(14-1960) (217) <u>H</u>

The Arthropod-Borne Viruses of Man and Other Animals
(14-1960) (261) <u>H</u>

Intramural Spread of Bacteria and Viruses in Human
Population
(14-1960) (43) <u>H</u>

The Epidemiology of Mouse Polyoma Virus Infection
(25-1961) (18) <u>B</u>

Smallpox and Related Poxvirus Infections in the
Simian Host
(25-1961) (459) <u>B</u>

Phage-Host Relationships in Some Genera of Medical
Significance
(15-1961) (153) <u>H</u>

Structure of Viruses
(15-1961) (219) <u>H</u>

Recent Experience with Antiviral Vaccines
(15-1961) (297) <u>H</u>

The Importance of Bacterial Viruses in Industry
Processes Esp. in the Dairy Industry
(4-1962) (51) <u>A</u>

Response of Cell and Organism to Infection with Avian
Tumor Viruses
(26-1962) (1) <u>B</u>

Viral Leukemias in Mice
(16-1962) (75) <u>H</u>

Genetics of Bacteriophage
(16-1962) (205) H

Cellular Resistance to Viral Infection, with Particular Reference to Endogenous Interferon
(27-1963) (72) B

Bacteriophage Reproduction
(17-1963) (87) H

The Interferons - Cellular Inhibitors of Viral
Infection
(17-1963) (285) H

Structure of Viral Nucleoproteins
(17-1963) (415) H

Malignant Transformation by Polyoma Virus
(17-1963) (167) H

Structure of Some Animal Viruses and Significance
of Their Components
(27-1963) (1) B

Harmful and Benefical Effects of Plant Viruses in
Insects
(17-1963) (495) H

Aspects of the Pathogenesis of Virus Diseases
(28-1964) (30) B

Enterovirus Entrance into Specific Host Cells and
Subsequent Alterations of Cell Protein and Nucleic
Acid Synthesis
(28-1964) (3) B

Current Progress in Virus Diseases - A Symposium
(28-1964) (367) B

Viral Infections of Domestic Animals
(18-1964) (269) H

The Genetics of Animal Viruses
(18-1964) (47) H

Kinetics of the Inactivation of Viruses
   (28-1964) (150) B

Viruses and Noah's Ark
   (29-1965) (1) B

Lactic Dehydrogenase Virus
   (29-1965) (173) B

Use of Ultrafiltration for Animal Virus Grouping
   (29-1965) (477) B

Recovery and Identification of Adenovirus in Infections of Infants and Children
   (29-1965) (487) B

Recovery and Identification of Human Myxoviruses
   (29-1965) (496) B

RNA Phages
   (19-1965) (455) H

Bacteriolysis
   (19-1965) (79) H

Host Controlled Modification of Bacteriophage
   (19-1965) (365) H

Chemotherapy of Cancer and Viral Infections
   (5-1965) (481) I

The Poxviruses
   (30-1966) (33) B

Multiplication of Measles Virus in Cell Cultures
   (30-1966) (152) B

Symposium on Replication of Viral Nucleic Acids
   (30-1966) (267) B

Pathogenesis of Rashes in Virus Diseases
   (30-1966) (739) B

The Classification of the Viruses
   (20-1966) (45) H

Biosynthetic Modifications Induced by DNA Animal
Viruses
   (20-1966) (189) H

Development and Evaluation of Antiviral and Antitumor Agents
   (6-1966) (483) I

Interferon
   (20-1966) (291) H

Epidemiological Aspects of Venezuelan Equine En-
cephalitis Virus Infections
   (31-1967) (65) B

Human Papova (Wart) Virus
   (31-1967) (110) B

Ultrastructure of Bacteriophages and Bacteriocins
   (31-1967) (230) B

Unusual Vectors of Plant Viruses
   (21-1967) (205) H

Virus Leukemia in the Mouse
   (21-1967) (529) H

Interferon Induction with Statolon in the Intact
Animal
   (31-1967) (132) B

Various Molecular Species of Interferon Induced
by Viral and Nonviral Agents
   (31-1967) (138) B

Cellular Resistance to Induction of Interferon
   (31-1967) (145) B

Production of Virus Vaccines
   (2-1967) (25) D #12

The Possible Role of Microorganisms and Viruses
in the Etiology of Chronic Degenerative Diseases
of Man
   (21-1967) (467) H

Recent Progress in Poxvirus Research
(32-1968) (127) B

Latent Virus Infections in Primate Tissues with
Special Reference to Simian Viruses
(32-1968) (185) B

First Step Transfer DNA of Bacteriophage T5
(32-1968) (227) B

Replication of RNA Viruses
(22-1968) (305) H

The Poxviruses
(22-1968) (359) H

The Oncogenic DNA Viruses: A Review of in Vitro
Transformation Studies
(22-1968) (391) H

Metabolism of Animal Cells Infected with Nuclear
DNA Viruses
(22-1968) (427) H

Lysogeny - The Integration Problem
(22-1968) (451) H

Bacteriophages, Their Biology and Industrial
Significance
(7-1968) (43) C

Applied Significance of Polyvalent Bacteriophage
(10-1968) (101) A

Antiviral Agents
(8-1968) (136) I

Filamentous Bacterial Viruses
(33-1969) (172) B

Death and Transfiguration of a Problem
(33-1969) (390) B

Mechanism of Perpetuation of Animal Viruses in Nature
(33-1969) (404) B

Thermophilic Bacteria and Bacteriophages
(3-1969) (83) E

Viral Studies
(9-1969) (148) I

Biological Activity of Bacteriophage Ghosts and
"Take Over" of Host Functions by Bacteriophage
(34-1970) (344) B

Regulation of Phage Development
(24-1970) (241) H

Reconstitution of Viruses
(24-1970) (463) H

Effect of Virus Infections on the Function of the
Immune System
(24-1970) (525) H

Myxovirus Ribonucleic Acids
(24-1970) (539) H

Large Scale Bacteriophage Production
(13-1970) (121) A

Genetics of Animal Viruses
(24-1970) (297) H

Newer Techniques in Virus Vaccine Production
(11-1970) (3) F

Expression of Animal Virus Genomes
(35-1971) (235) B

Viruses with Segmented RNA Genomes: Multiplication
of Influenza Versus Reovirus
(35-1971) (250) B

Comparative Virology of Primates
(35-1971) (310) B

Survey of Numerical Techniques for Grouping
(25-1971) (379) D

Role of Viruses as Causes of Congenital Defects
(25-1971) (255) H

Mechanism of Cell Transformation by RNA Tumor
Viruses
(25-1971) (609) H

Interferon Induction and Action
(25-1971) (333) H

Mechanisms of Virus Pathogenecity
(36-1972) (291) B

Rhinoviruses
(26-1972) (503) H

RNA Virus Gene Expression and Its Control
(26-1972) (467) H

Production of Virus Vaccines in Human Diploid Cell
Strains
(8-1973) (28) D #2

Monkeypox Virus
(37-1973) (1) B

Viral Teratology
(37-1973) (19) B

Early Events in Cell-Animal Virus Interaction
(37-1973) (103) B

VITAMINS

Microbial Synthesis of Cobamines
(1-1959) (87) A

Production and Biosynthesis of Riboflavin in Microorganisms
(1-1959) (137) C

The Microbiological Production of Vitamin B12 and
  Sulphide
  (2-1960) (27) C

The Biochemistry of the Vitamin B12 Fermentation
  (5-1964) (151) C

Microbial Carotenogenesis
  (7-1965) (1) A

The Biosynthesis and Function of Carotenoid
  Pigments in Microorganisms
  (19-1965) (163) H

Vitamin B12 from Sewage Sludge
  (4-1969) (25) D #12

Vitamin B12 Isolation
  (4-1969) (35) D #12

Fermentation Processes Employed in Vitamin C
  Syntheses
  (12-1970) (11) A

Microbial Biosynthesis of B12 Like Compounds
  (24-1970) (159) H

Microbial Carotenoids
  (26-1972) (225) H

Riboflavin Oversynthesis
  (26-1972) (369) H

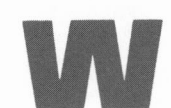

WASTE DISPOSAL AND WATER TREATMENT

Newer Aspects of Waste Treatment
    (2-1960) (1) A

Problems in Water Microbiology
    (3-1962) (306) F

Purification and Sanitary Control of Water
    (16-1962) (127) H

Waste Treatment
    (4-1963) (93) F

Microbial Aspects of Water Pollution Control
    (6-1964) (119) A

Biologically Hard and Trace Contaminants of Natural
    Waters
    (4-1964) (53) F

The Ecological Approach to the Study of Activated
    Sludge
    (8-1966) (77) A

Control of Bacteria in Nondomestic Water Supplies
(8-1966) (105) A

The Presence of Human Enteric Viruses in Sewage and
Their Removal by Conventional Sewage Treatment
Methods
(8-1966) (145) A

An Introduction to the Activated Sludge Process
(1-1966) (15) D

Trends in Sewage Purification Equipment, Part 1
(1-1966) (151) D

Trends in Sewage Purification Equipment, Part 2
(1-1966) (244) D

Activated Sludge Plant Design Problems
(1-1966) (257) D

Wet Air Oxidation of Sewage Sludge
(1-1966) (329) D

Biological Treatment of Industrial Waste
(1-1966) (385) D

Plastics in Waste Treatment, Part 1
(1-1966) (483) D

Waste Waters - The Future
(1-1966) (84) D

Methanogenesis and Anaerobic Treatment of Waste
- Symposium
(7-1966) (131) F

Microbiology of Waste Waters
(20-1966) (319) H

Plastics in Waste Treatment, Part 2
(2-1967) (31) D #1

Organic Matter in Liquid Wastes
(2-1967) (11) D #2

International Water Pollution Research
(2-1967) (27) D #2

Large Volume Respirometers with Particular Reference to Waste-Treatment
(6-1967) (1414) C

Sludge Dewatering Treatment
(2-1967) (17) D #3

Anaerobic Fermentation of Sewage Sludge
(2-1967) (11) D #8

Cannery Effluent Problems
(2-1967) (7) D #4

Aspects of the Activated Sludge Processes
(2-1967) (39) D #10

Temperature Relationships in Municipal Composting
(2-1967) (44) D #6

Effluent Purification from Potato Chip Manufacture
(2-1967) (45) D #7

Organic Matter in Liquid Wastes
(2-1967) (11) D #2

Anaerobic Sludge Digestion
(2-1967) (52) D #11

Anaerobic Sludge Digestion (Part 2)
(2-1967) (17) D #12

Bulking of Activated Sludge
(9-1967) (185) A

Separation Technique - Sludge Dewatering
(2-1967) (34) D #9

Incineration of Sewage Sludge
(3-1968) (60) D #4

Contact Stabilization
(3-1968) (35) D #1

Decanters for Sludge Dewatering
    (5-1970) (19) <u>D</u> #1

R & D in Waste Water Treatment
    (5-1970) (23) <u>D</u> #1

Shallow Depth Settling
    (5-1970) (27) <u>D</u> #1

Tertiary Effluent Demineralization
    (5-1970) (31) <u>D</u> #1

Coilfilter for Sewage Treatment
    (5-1970) (49) <u>D</u> #1

Vapour Incineration
    (5-1970) (54) <u>D</u> #1

Centrifuges in Sewage Treatment
    (5-1970) (51) <u>D</u> #1

Polymers in Water Treatment
    (5-1970) (28) <u>D</u> #2

Potato Processing Waste
    (5-1970) (65) <u>D</u> #3

Solid State Control for Water Treatment
    (5-1970) (33) <u>D</u> #3

Effects of Organic Wastes on Rivers
    (5-1970) (44) <u>D</u> #4

Microbiological Utilization of Sulfite Liquor
    (5-1970) (35) <u>D</u> #6

Local Authority - And Industrial Effluents
    (5-1970) (53) <u>D</u> #6

Deodorization of Industrial Waste Water
    (5-1970) (59) <u>D</u> #6

Biochemical Reduction of Waste
    (5-1970) (47) <u>D</u> #7

Effluent Treatment in Process Industries
(5-1970) (52) D #9

Pasteurization and Sterilization of Sludges
(5-1970) (44) D #9

Trends in Sewage Treatment
(6-1971) (15) D #1

Vacuum Filtration of Sludge
(6-1971) (21) D #1

Advances in Multihearth Incineration
(6-1971) (27) D #1

Immedium Filter in Tertiary Treatment
(6-1971) (33) D #1

Waste Disposal Techniques
(6-1971) (49) D #1

Water and Protein Reclamation from Sewage
(6-1971) (50) D #1

Economical Solution to Water Pollution
(6-1971) (45) D #3

Microbiological Aspects of Seawater Pollution
(12-1971) (109) F

Anaerobic Digestion in Biological Waste Treatment
(9-1971) (155) C

Water Treatment - A Review
(7-1972) (13) D #1

Automated Analysis of Effluent
(7-1972) (16) D #1

Waste Treatment for Small Communities
(7-1972) (18) D #1

Mechanical Aeration
(7-1972) (23) D #1

Fermentation of Pollutants
    (7-1972) (27) D #1

Automation of an Activated Sludge Plant
    (7-1972) (17) D #2

Phosphorous Removal from Sewage
    (7-1972) (17) D #6

Treatment of Livestock Wastes
    (7-1972) (21) D #6

Centrifugal Dewatering of Sludges
    (7-1972) (27) D #6

Microbial Aspects of Solid Wastes Disposal
    (13-1972) (9) F

Automation of an Activated Sludge Plant - 2
    (7-1972) (21) D #9

Problems of Odour
    (7-1972) (17) D #11

Waste Recovery by Microorganisms
    (7-1972) (21) D #11

Sludge Treatment - The Current Trends
    (8-1973) (11) D #1

Activated Sludge - Industrial Case History
    (8-1973) (11) D #1

The Bacteriology of Anaerobic Sewage Digestion
    (8-1973) (19) D #1

Developments in Sludge and Waste Incineration
    (8-1973) (27) D #1

The Cyclone Furnace for Waste
    (8-1973) (29) D #1

Microbiology in the Aerobic Treatment of Farm Waste
    (8-1973) (28) D #3

Detectors for Measurement of Water Pollution
   (8-1973) (31) D #3

Sludge Thickening by Flotation
   (8-1973) (26) D #5

Physical Chemical Treatment of Sewage in the US
   (8-1973) (11) D #6

Automatic Samplers for Sewage and Effluents
   (8-1973) (15) D #6

Electrochemical Process for Effluent
   (8-1973) (19) D #6

WINERY OPERATIONS

Bacterial Spoilage of Wine
   (1-1966) (265) D

Table Wine Manufacture
   (2-1967) (5) D #1

Winemaking by Continuous Fermentation
   (2-1967) (44) D #12

The Malo-Lactic Fermentation
   (9-1967) (235) A

Separation Techniques - Wine
   (2-1967) (32) D #9

Sherry Manufacture
   (3-1968) (41) D #2

Flor Yeasts in Sherry
   (3-1968) (11) D #7

Microbiology of Winemaking
   (22-1968) (323) H

Aspects of Wine Maturation
   (3-1968) (43) D̲ #12

The Manufacture of Port
   (7-1972) (27) D̲ #10

Volatile Aroma Components of Wines and Other
  Fermented Beverages
   (15-1972) (75) A̲

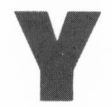

YEAST

Recent Research on the Yeasts
(3-1961) (1) C

The Cell Walls of Yeast
(17-1963) (15) H

Uses and Products of Yeasts and Yeast-Like
Fungi
(7-1965) (225) A

Hybridization of Yeasts
(1-1966) (25) D

Processing Brewers Yeast
(1-1966) (313) D

Flocculation of Brewers Yeast
(1-1966) (489) D

Yeast Genetics
(20-1966) (151) H

Aspects of Commercial Yeast Production
(2-1967) (41) D #3

Infection Control in Yeast Factories and Breweries
    (2-1967) (11) D #12

Yeast as a Source of Biochemicals
    (3-1968) (59) D #8

Production of Polyhydric Alcohols by Yeasts
    (7-1968) (1) C

Production of Brewers Yeast
    (3-1968) (21) D #12

Identification of Yeasts
    (3-1968) (32) D #5

Manufacture of Bakers Yeast
    (3-1968) (45) D #7

Molecular Basis of Mating in the Yeast Hansenula
  wingei
    (32-1968) (139) B

Budding of Yeast Cells, Their Scars and Aging
    (2-1968) (143) E

Pure Yeast Cultures in Brewing
    (5-1970) (15) D #4

Differentiation of Commercial Yeasts
    (5-1970) (29) D #4

Yeast Autolysis
    (5-1970) (50) D #5

Thermophilic Enteric Yeasts
    (25-1971) (49) H

SECTION III - MICROBIOLOGICAL JOURNALS AND ABSTRACT SERVICES

This section contains a listing of 30 of the more prominent journals and abstracting services available to the industrial microbiologist. The countries represented in the journal listing include Canada, Czechoslovakia, England, India, France, Japan and the United States. The four abstract services cited are prepared from papers in over 20 languages.

All subscription prices quoted are those charged nonmembers. Member subscriptions are usually considerably less costly.

AGRICULTURAL AND BIOLOGICAL CHEMISTRY - A Monthly Publication of the Agricultural Chemical Society of Japan. Japan Publications Trading Co., Inc. 175 Fifth Avenue, New York, N. Y. 10010

Organization

A	Analytical Chemistry
B	Organic Chemistry
C	Biological Chemistry
D	Food and Nutrition
E	Microbiology and Fermentation Industry
F	Pesticides
G	Soil and Fertilizer

Subscription Price - $40.00/yr.

ANNALES D'IMMUNOLOGIE - Masson Et Cie Editeurs - 120, Boulevard Saint-Germain, Paris, VIe. Quarterly Organe de la Societe Francoise de Microbiologie. Collection Des Annales De L'Institute Pasteur.

ANNALES DE MICROBIOLOGIE - Masson Et Cie Editeurs - 120, Boulevard Saint-Germain, Paris, VIe. Monthly Organe de la Societe Francoise de Microbiologie. Collection Des Annales De L'Institut Pasteur.

Organization

I	Microbiologie Generale. Physiologie et Genetique Bacteriennes
II	Microbiologie Medicale
III	Microbiologie Appliquee
IV	Virologie

ANTIMICROBIAL AGENTS AND CHEMOTHERAPY - A Monthly Production of the American Society for Microbiology. ASM Publications Office, 1913 I Street, N. W., Washington, D. C. 20006.

Subscription Price - $40.00/year.

APPLIED MICROBIOLOGY - A Monthly Production of the American Society for Microbiology, ASM Publications Office, 1913 I Street, N. W., Washington, D. C. 20006.

Organization

A	Clinical Microbiology and Immunology
B	Virology and Viral Immunology
C	Food Microbiology and Toxicology
D	Ecology
E	Metabolism and End Products
F	Disinfectants

Subscription Price - $60.00/year.

BACTERIOLOGICAL REVIEWS - A Quarterly Production of the
American Society for Microbiology (March, June, September,
and December). ASM Publications Office, 1913 I Street,
N. W., Washington, D. C. 20006.

Subscription Price - $12.00/year.

BIOTECHNOLOGY AND BIOENGINEERING - Editor Elmer L. Gaden,
Jr., Published Bimonthly by John Wiley and Sons, Inc.
605 3rd Avenue, New York, N. Y. 10016.

Subscription Price - $75.00/year.

CANADIAN JOURNAL OF MICROBIOLOGY - Published Monthly by the
National Research Council of Canada, Ottawa.

Organization

A	General
B	Immunology and Immunochemistry
C	Infection and Immunity
D	Physiology
E	Virology

Subscription Price - $12.00/year.

FOLIA MICROBIOLOGICA - Distributed by Academia, Publishing
House of Czechoslovak Academy of Sciences, Vodickova 40,
11229 Praha 1-Noce Mesto, Czechoslovakia. Published
Bimonthly.

HINDUSTAN ANTIBIOTICS BULLETIN - Published Quarterly by
Hindustan Antibiotics Ltd. Pimpri, Poona-18 India.

Each issue contains an Antibiotics Literature Index
arranged under the following headings:

General
New Antibiotics
Antibiotic Producing Organisms
Production
Pharmaceutics

Chemistry
Biochemical Studies
Molecular Biology
Microbiology
Pharmacology
Therapeutics
Veterinary Medicine
Non-Pharmaceutical Uses.

Subscription Price - $4.00/year.

INFECTION AND IMMUNITY - A Monthly Production of the American Society for Microbiology, ASM Publications Office, 1913 I Street, N. W., Washington, D. C. 20006.

Organization

A   Bacterial and Mycotic Infections
B   Viral Infections
C   Pathogenic Mechanisms, Ecology and Epidemiology
D   Immunology

Subscription Price - $40.00/year.

INTERNATIONAL JOURNAL OF SYSTEMATIC BACTERIOLOGY - A Quarterly Production of the American Society for Microbiology, ASM Publications Office, 1913 I Street, N. W., Washington, D. C. 20006.

Subscription Price - $8.00/year.

JAPANESE JOURNAL OF MICROBIOLOGY - Published Bimonthly by Japan Bacteriological Society and Society of Japanese Virologists. Distributor for USA and Canada is Springer-Verlag New York, Inc., 175 5th Avenue, New York, N. Y. 10010.

Subscription Price is ¥ 10,800/year.

JOURNAL OF ANTIBIOTICS, THE - A Monthly Journal Published
by Japan Antibiotics Research Association, Editorial
Office - Japan Antibiotics Research Association, 2-20-8,
Kamiosaki, Shinagawa, Tokyo, Japan.

Subscription Price - $30.00/year.

JOURNAL OF APPLIED BACTERIOLOGY, THE - Published 4 Times
Per Year by the Society for Applied Bacteriology. Academic Press, Inc., 111 5th Avenue, New York, N. Y. 10003.

Subscription Price $29.70 plus $1.95 postage.

JOURNAL OF BACTERIOLOGY - A Monthly Production of the American Society for Microbiology, ASM Publications Office,
1913 I Street, N. W., Washington, D. C. 20006.

Organization

A	Morphology and Ultrastructure
B	Genetics and Molecular Biology
C	Physiology and Metabolism
D	Enzymology

Subscription Price - $75.00/year.

JOURNAL OF FERMENTATION TECHNOLOGY - Monthly Journal of
the Society of Fermentation Technology of Japan, Faculty
of Engineering, Osaka University, Yamada Kami, Suita,
Osaka 565 Japan. Feb., April, June, August, October,
and December Issues are in English. Other Months are in
Japanese with English Abstracts.

Subscription Price - $25.00/year.

JOURNAL OF GENERAL MICROBIOLOGY, THE - Published Monthly for
the Society for General Microbiology. Cambridge University Press, 32 East 57th Street, New York, N. Y. 10022.

Organization

A   Physiology and Growth
B   Biochemistry
C   Genetics and Molecular Biology
D   Ecology
E   Taxonomy
F   Short Communication

Subscription Price - $26.50/volume.

JOURNAL OF GENERAL VIROLOGY - Published Monthly for the
Society for General Microbiology, Cambridge University
Press, 32 East 57th Street, New York, N. Y.   10022.

Subscription Price - $26.50/volume.

JOURNAL OF IMMUNOLOGY, THE - Monthly Publication of the
American Association of Immunologists. Published by
Williams and Wilkins Co., Baltimore, Md.

Organization

A   Cellular Immunology
B   Immunochemistry
C   Immunogenetics and Transplantation
D   Immunopathology
E   Viral and Microbial Immunology
F   Communication

Subscription Price - $48.00/year.

JOURNAL OF INFECTIOUS DISEASES, THE - Monthly Publication of
the Infectious Diseases Society of America. Published by
the University of Chicago Press, Chicago, Ill. 60637.
Covers Medical Microbiology, Clinical Immunology and Epidemiology.

Subscription Price - $50.00/year.

JOURNAL OF MEDICAL MICROBIOLOGY - Published Quarterly by Longman Group Limited, Journals Division, 43-45 Annandale Street, Edinburgh EH74AT, England. An Official Journal of the Pathological Society of Great Britain and Ireland.

Subscription Price - $24.00/year.

JOURNAL OF VIROLOGY - A Monthly Publication of the American Society for Microbiology - ASM Publications Office, 1913 I Street, N. W., Washington, D. C. 20006.

Organization

A	Animal Viruses
B	Bacterial Viruses
C	Plant Viruses

Subscription Price - $40.00/year.

MICROBIOLOGICAL ABSTRACTS - Section A - Industrial and Applied Microbiology. (10,000 Abstracts per Annum Prepared from Papers in 20 Languages.) Published by Information Retrieval Limited, 1 Falconberg Court, London W1V5FG, England.

MICROBIOLOGICAL ABSTRACTS - Section B - Bacteriology. (10,000 Abstracts per Annum Prepared from Papers in 20 Languages.) Published by Information Retrieval Limited, 1 Falconberg Court, London W1V5FG, England.

MICROBIOLOGICAL ABSTRACTS - Section C - Algology, Mycology and Protozoalogy. (8,000 Abstracts per Annum Prepared from Papers in 20 Languages.) Published by Information Retrieval Limited, 1 Falconberg Court, London W1V5FG, England.

MYCOLOGIA - Published Bimonthly for The New York Botanical Garden, Lancaster, Pa. 17604. Official Organ of the Mycological Society of America.

Subscription Price - $20.00/year.

PROCESS BIOCHEMISTRY - Consulting Editor: I. L. Hepner,
Editor: Rosemary Parker, Publisher: Morgan-Grampian Ltd.,
Morgan Grampian House, 30 Calderwood Street, Woolwich,
London SE 18 6 QH. Monthly Publication Covering the Food,
Brewing, Water and Effluent Treatment, Pharmaceutical and
Allied Biochemical Industries.

Subscription Price - £ 10/Annum.

VIRAL ABSTRACTS - Published by Information Retrieval Limited,
1 Falconberg Court, London W1V5FG, England. (7,000 Abstracts per Annum Prepared from Papers in 20 Languages.)

VIROLOGY - Published Monthly by Academic Press, Inc., 111
5th Avenue, New York, N. Y. 10003.

Subscription Price - $25.00/volume.

SECTION IV - MEETINGS AND COURSES

Another important source of current information is
obtained from meetings that are held -- both national and
international. In most cases the abstracts of the papers
presented in the sessions are printed and available at
the time of the meeting.

A. NATIONAL MEETINGS

American Society for Microbiology

Future Meetings: 1974 - Chicago, May 12-17
1975 - New York, April 27 - May 2

Papers are abstracted in The Abstracts of the
Annual Meeting of the American Society for
Microbiology

Interscience Conference on Antimicrobial Agents and Chemotherapy

Future Meetings: 1974 - San Francisco, Sept. 11-13
Meetings are held annually during the Fall and
are sponsored by the American Society for Microbiology.

Papers are abstracted in The Program and Abstracts
of the Interscience Conference on Antimicrobial
Agents and Chemotherapy.

American Chemical Society - Division of Microbial Chemistry and Technology

Future Meetings: 1974 - Atlantic City, Sept. 8-13
                   1975 - Chicago, Aug. 24-29
                   1976 - San Francisco, Aug. 29-Sept. 3
                   1977 - Chicago, Aug. 28-Sept. 2
                   1978 - Miami Beach, Sept. 10-15
                   1979 - Houston, Sept. 9-14
                   1980 - San Francisco, Aug. 24-29

Papers are abstracted in Abstracts of Papers.

Society for Industrial Microbiology

Meetings are held annually during the fall.

Proceedings of the annual meeting are published in
Developments in Industrial Microbiology.

B.   INTERNATIONAL MEETINGS

International Congress for Microbiology

The last meeting (i.e., the Tenth Congress) was
held in Mexico City in 1970.

The papers presented at the meeting were published
in Recent Advances in Microbiology. Abstracts
were also available at the meeting.

International Fermentation Symposium

The 3rd International Symposium was held in 1968 in New Brunswick, N.J.

The papers presented at the meeting were published in Fermentation Advances.

The 4th International Symposium was held in 1972 in Kyoto, Japan.

The papers presented at the meeting were published in Fermentation Technology Today.

Abstracts were also available at both meetings.

C. COURSES

Fermentation Technology

Massachusetts Institute of Technology, Cambridge, Massachusetts.

The 1973 summer session covered the following subjects:

Growth and Metabolism
Coordination of Microbial Metabolism
Biosynthesis of Metabolites
Power Requirements in Fermentation Vessels
Mass Transfer in Fermentation Vessels
Translation to Differing Operating Scales
Instrumentation and Control of Fermentation Processes
Theory, Application and Techniques of Continuous
    Culture
Enzyme Science, Technology and Engineering
Recovery Processes
Media and Air Sterilization

Cost: $375

Address inquiries to Professor Daniel I. C. Wang,
Department of Nutrition and Food Science.

Enzyme Engineering

Engineering Foundation Conferences, Engineering
Foundation, 345 East 47 Street, New York,
N. Y. 10017

The 1971 Conference was held August 9-13 in Henniker,
New Hampshire and the proceedings were published
in Enzyme Engineering.

The 1973 Conference was held August 5-10 in Henniker,
New Hampshire. The proceedings are to be pub-
lished by Interscience Publishers, a division of
John Wiley and Sons. Subjects covered in this
Conference include the following:

Developments in Enzyme Technology since 1971
New Purification Techniques
New Immobilization Techniques and Supports
Multiple Enzyme Immobilization and Multienzyme
    Systems. Physical Methods for Examining
    Immobilized Enzymes
Use of Immobilized Coenzymes
Reactor Design
Industrial Processes Using Enzymes
Commercial Aspects of Enzymes
New Applications of Enzymes

Cost $160